Organic Mental Disease

Organic Mental Disease

Frank R. Freemon, M.D.
Neurology Service
Nashville Veterans Administration Hospital
and
Department of Neurology
Vanderbilt University School of Medicine, Nashville

MTP PRESS LIMITED
International Medical Publishers

Published in the UK and Europe by
MTP Press Limited
Falcon House
Lancaster, England

Published in the US by
SPECTRUM PUBLICATIONS, INC.
175-20 Wexford Terrace
Jamaica, N.Y. 11432

Softcover reprint of the hardcover 1st edition 1981

ISBN-13: 978-94-011-7288-2 e-ISBN-13: 978-94-011-7286-8
DOI: 10.1007/978-94-011-7286-8

To my wife LINDA

Preface

This book is written for the clinician who cares for adult patients with organic mental disease—with dysfunction of the brain producing mental symptoms. It should be read from cover to cover in order to get an overview of the field, if this misshapen mass of art, knowledge, tradition, and myth can be called a field. Since organic mental patients, often depressed themselves, sometimes induce depression in their physicians, I have interspersed a few amusing anecdotes and outrageous analogies to raise morale. This book is not intended to be a step-by-step cookbook, but rather to discuss principles which each practitioner can adapt to his own patient population. Nor is it intended to be an encyclopedic reference work, although sufficient quotation to the medical literature should permit the interested reader to plunge to whatever depth he desires.

The present editorial custom in the United States requires combined male and female pronouns. According to this fad, the previous paragraph should have ended "he or she desires" or "he/she desires." With a few exceptions, men and women suffer organic mental disease with equal frequency and equal severity, therefore all male pronouns and adjectives used in this book are intended to be neuter. When I refer to the patient's spouse as "his wife," please imagine that half the time it reads "her husband."

The author thanks his excellent typists, Beth Gehrke and Elizabeth Jaeckle. He also acknowledges the courtesy of the following copyright holders for permission to reproduce their works: The American Physiological Society for Figure 1 in the first chapter (from Allen and Tsukahara, *Physiological Reviews*, 1974), Atheneum Publishers for Eric Hodgins description of his stroke (Hodgins, *Episode*, 1963), and Richard Marek Publishers for Dr. Samuel Shem's description of a particularly difficult organic mental disease patient (Shem, *House of God*, 1978). Also, I am required by V.A. regulations (circular 10-79-61) to acknowledge that my research mentioned in this book was "supported by the Veterans Administration."

Frank R. Freemon, M.D.

Contents

Chapter 1

Localization of Mental Function

INTRODUCTION

This book is directed at physicians who evaluate and treat patients with organic mental disease—patients with changes in consciousness, thinking, emotion, or behavior associated with histopathological changes in central nervous tissue. Many, if not most, physicians approach these patients with certain underlying assumptions about the relationship of brain to mind. Failure to recognize these unconscious assumptions is the greatest single impediment to understanding organic mental dysfunction and to properly and humanely treating the many people who suffer from these disorders.

Most people accept this axiom: Diseases that affect the brain often affect the mind also. If the reader does not now believe this, he certainly will upon concluding this book. This is not to say that all brain diseases affect the mind; a cerebellar tumor can cause severe motor deficits, but mental abilities are completely unaffected. Note also, that not everyone accepts the converse; diseases which affect the mind, such as depression, do not cause histopathologic changes in brain.

Since most people accept this axiom, what is the problem? The problem is a practical one; a problem of patient management, physician responsibility, and the legal determination of the patient's right to determine his own fate. The neurologist disregards the patient's unrealistic or paranoid concepts; he feels that the patient's disease must receive medical and/or surgical therapy, then his responsibility ends. The psychiatrist, in turn, feels incompetent in the evaluation of organic disease and he too withdraws.

The problem can be exemplified by an actual case. A patient has cancer of the lung, metastatic to the brain. He has undergone a severe personality change; his behavior has become childish and dependent. When he speaks to others he likes to hold tight to their hand and arm. He speaks in a somewhat dysarthric voice, but the words flow very quickly. His thoughts, although jumbled with extraneous observations, always return to worries about his burial. He knows he has a malignant tumor and will die soon. The patient sometimes wants to be buried in the family plot beside his twin sister, and sometimes requests burial in another town where his wife intends to be buried with her family. All his waking hours are spent talking about burial to his brother, who has power of attorney, and his wife, who is the next of kin and will have disposition over his final remains. When consulted by the family, the psychiatrist says it is a neurologic problem, a brain tumor, and his involvement is therefore limited to a determination of incompetency for legal purposes. The neurologist says that his examination shows periods of disorientation and that the patient is not responsible for what he says; his exact words to the family were, "that's just the tumor talking now." Meanwhile, the family, caught between specialists, struggles along without medical help or any real counseling. Everyone involved, including the patient, hopes the tumor grows rapidly enough to conclude this confusion.

The philosophic dogma of dualism—of the two separate worlds of insubstantial mind and physical brain—produces a dual approach to the sick person. The psychiatrist, despite his humorous appellation of "head shrinker," treats only disorders of the mind; the neurologist and neurosurgeon treat brain diseases. The patient with organic mental disease falls helplessly between the two.

RELATIONSHIPS BETWEEN BRAIN AND MIND

The busy clinician or overwhelmed student feels he has little time to devote to philosophic issues. We must do something *now* about the person who used to flirt with the idea of suicide but has just bought a gun. The practical consequences of the dualistic mind/brain assumptions that unconsciously guide our clinical behavior are so great, however, that a very brief review of some of the philosophic issues is warranted.

While there is little doubt that events in the neural world and events in the mental world are somehow related, many argue about the direction and degree of that relationship. Some hold that the brain is a transducer for the mind. Mental activity goes on with or without a brain; but, when the mind wants to effect a change in the real world, it changes neural processes in order to produce muscular movements which make the necessary manipulations. Others hold that consciousness is an epiphenomenon; brain activities generate mental functions, but neural events in the brain continue to direct behavior regardless of what mental activity is generated. More complex relationships have also been posited. Perhaps a neural event generates a mental one which, in turn, generates another neural event, and so on (Wilson, 1976). Abnormalities of function in the mental sphere will be reflected in neural changes and vice versa. Observe that these formulations attempt to identify a relationship and the direction of that relationship, but make no effort to examine the mechanism by which a physical event in an anatomical structure can change or be changed by a nonphysical mental event.

Figure 1 exemplifies how the mind/brain dichotomy can intrude into a purely neurological formulation. Allen and Tsukahara (1974) compare the neural mechanism that initiates and directs movements to a computer program. Their summary diagram includes the "idea" of the movement, which somehow changes neural activity in association cortex to trigger off the movement mechanism. Most neuroscientists and neurological clinicians have unspoken assumptions about the mental activities behind, initiating, or corresponding to neural activities, but few picture this relationship as clearly as Allen and Tsukahara have.

If we temporarily put aside the question of causality and limit ourselves to examinations of relationship alone, we encounter basic agreement among all

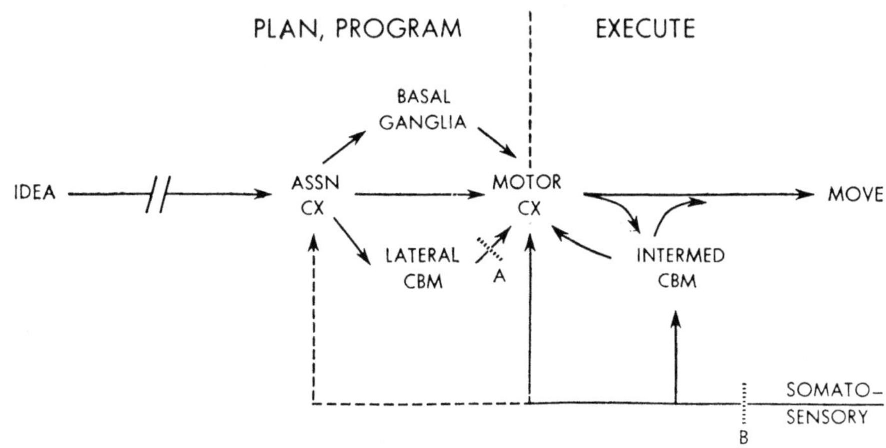

Figure 1: This figure is reproduced from the review article by Allen and Tsukahara (1974) on how the brain controls movement. The authors include the "idea" which initiates the neural mechanism. The broken line between the idea and association cortex symbolizes the enigma of this mental to physical transformation. Copyright © American Physiological Association.

factions, with certain reservations about the initiating element—the will or the "ghost in the machine." The basic accepted relationship gōes under the rubric of the mind/brain identity theory (Borst, 1970), the psychoneural identity hypothesis (Feigl, 1967), or the psycho(neural) event identity thesis (Globus, 1973), and accepts the notion that events in the mental world are precisely identical with events in the brain.

Some philosophers invoke the mathematical concept of isomorphism. This concept relates two series of elements to each other by certain specific laws. The two systems are isomorphic if they have the same number of elements and if certain specified transformations of the elements produce the same effects. For example, the entire series of positive integrers is isomorphic to the series of even positive digits, using the transformations of addition and subtraction. At first, one might think that this could not be so, that the full series of integers would be twice as large as the series of even integers only. Actually, both contain an infinite number of elements. If one arranges the series in ascending order and adds the second and third elements, one obtains the fifth (2+3=5, 4+6=10). This is true for all elements using the transformations of addition and subtraction. Various mathematical techniques are used to prove that one series is isomorphic to another.

Mathematicians have great fun finding two systems which have little apparent relationship to one another but which, when expressed mathematically, are isomorphic to one another. For example, one might be able to prove that the Shakespearean ages of man is a system isomorphic to the colors of the rainbow, using the transformations of moving in one direction (birth to death, violet to red) and in the opposite direction. So, it is hypothesized that the brain consists of a series of elements, perhaps neurons, which interact with each other, perhaps by synaptic contact, and this system is isomorphic to a mental system of even more poorly defined elements and interactions.

This book recommends that individuals involved with organic mental disease patients use the working model of brain function, termed psychoneural identity or brain/mind isomorphism. This model holds that histopathological lesions in certain parts of the brain interfere with mental processes. The characteristics of the mental dysfunction predict the location and, sometimes, the type of underlying disease process. Furthermore, to say that a certain type of lession "causes" a certain type of behavior is an oversimplification—perhaps necessary for rapid communication, but not always fair to the patient. Before the disease began, the patient's brain generated (or, more formally, was associated with) a certain type of behavior. This could be studied objectively by external observors, but the patient-to-be felt that his behavior was under his own control. When the disease damages the brain, according to the model, the mind is also "damaged," or, in more common terms, the patient's mental dysfunction becomes apparent. The patient's mind, although impaired, is still his own.

To use an analogy, imagine a B-29 with two engines destroyed by German Messerschmitt fighters. The pilot is working frantically to stabilize the plane on its remaining two engines and return to England. He is still in some measure of control. He can turn the plane to the left or right, although he has much greater difficulty than he had on the way to Germany and he may resort to some piloting tricks he has never had to use before. Unless or until the plane crashes, the difference between a dysfunctioning B-29 and one functioning normally is a difference of degree, not a dichotomy of control. Although the plane has been damaged, its control has not been taken from the pilot.

So it is with the patient with organic mental disease. His mental abilities are different, generally less than normal, yet he still feels in control of his own destiny. He is prone to the same emotional upsets as are people with undamaged brains; in fact he may be more so because his decreased brain function may mean that he is less capable of complex mental defense mechanisms and must, therefore, revert to more primitive, possibly less adaptive, mental defenses. From a practical point of view, this model means that the problems of each organic mental patient must be overcome with a two-pronged attack. The basic underlying disease must receive medical or neurosurgical therapy; simultaneously, the patient's emotional problems should receive appropriate treatment. The patient usually has much better insight into his illness than many traditional psychiatric patients and is amenable to supportive psychotherapy. In addition, he may benefit from psychiatric pharmacological treatment; if he is depressed he may need treatment with tricyclic antidepressants, for example. In the terms of the mind/brain dichotomist, the damaged brain responds to pharmacologic therapy in much the same way as does the undamaged one, with certain important exceptions. In the view of the organic psychiatrist, a brain working improperly because of a histopathologic lesion responds to pharmacologic therapy much as the brain with a biochemical imbalance does.

Examples of the correct application of this philosophy include the use of electroshock therapy in the treatment of pharmacologically unresponsive depression in a patient with brain tumor (Dressler and Folk, 1975) and the use of several psychiatric therapies to overcome severe emotional disturbance in a mentally retarded patient with Down's syndrome (Satten and Singer, 1979). An example of the opposing, and in my opinion incorrect, view is the assertion of Pribram (1973), who suggests that "we limit direct therapeutic brain manipulation to those patients whose brains have been shown to be abnormal in function, and that we resort to behavioral means to treat those people for whom we have been able to demonstrate only behavioral abnormalities." Further examples of the practical problems which derive from the philosophical position which completely separates mental and brain function are discussed by Schoenberg and his colleagues (1978).

CEREBRAL LOCALIZATION OF MENTAL FUNCTION

Ancient Times

Knowledge of a relationship between mind and brain (or perhaps better in this context, behavior and intracranial contents) extends back to before recorded history, when early man observed the results of head injuries. The oldest compilation of medical observations, the Egyptian papyri collected and translated by Edwin Smith, records paralysis after head injury. These may be interpreted to suggest that the ancient Egyptians knew that one side of the brain controls the opposite side of the body. The early Greeks, particularly Aristotle, believed that control of emotions resided in the heart. Presumably, this false premise arose from an over-dependence on introspection as a source of data. Galen observed the result of combat injuries to the head and chest, especially in Roman gladiators, and correctly discounted this concept.

The presumed localization of emotions to the heart continues to be subscribed to, however. A recent newspaper article related the observations of a young woman who discovered many of the personality traits of her dead husband in the man who had received her husband's heart in transplatation. Heart transplantation is the subject of a not-so-funny joke about heart and personality: "Today the first successful transplant of a chimpanzee heart into man has been accomplished. The patient is doing well except for an uncontrollable desire to pick lice out of his wife's hair." If the reader thinks he is above these primitive concepts of emotional localization, he should study the shape of the missive given to his spouse next Valentine's Day.

Following Galen's lead, medical scientists up until the eighteenth century generally considered all thoughts and emotions to originate or reside within the brain. By analogy to hydraulic systems, it was thought that the brain influenced behavior by the passage of fluid. It was known that fluid resided within the brain ventricles and the spinal canal. Somehow, mental activity shifted this fluid down hollow neural tubules to fill the muscles which expanded during contraction. This idea seems a bit fanciful but is not really too different from the modern model, except that electricity has replaced hydraulic fluid. A good deal of circumstantial evidence from rapid exsanguination to chronic post-nasal drip related changes in body fluids to disease states and it was easy to imagine how disease processes could affect normal hydraulic nervous function. Different theories, completely without basis, attributed different mental abilities to various ventricular spaces. The first man to attribute psychological function to actual brain tissue, and to propose a method to localize that function to various portions of the brain was Franz Joseph Gall.

Phrenology

The saga of phrenology includes the ridiculous and the sublime. The close of the nineteenth century saw phrenology "practiced" by a group of glib semi-charlatans who predicted personality from bumps on the head. Prominent citizens submitted to a "phrenological examination" in order to determine their mental abilities and emotional foibles. Figure 2, from a phrenological journal of this period, reproduces the "official" report on the Chinese ambassador to the United States. Phrenology at the end of the nineteenth century might be compared to astrology at the close of the twentieth century, predicting personal qualities by date of birth. Phrenology died an atrophic death, as will astrology, but it began as an exciting hypothesis of mental function. Its subsequent decline and degradation obscures its initial brilliance, and causes modern neuroscientists to deny their historical origins.

Do all theoretical systems begin with a single observation? When he was in grammar school, about the year 1770, Franz Joseph Gall noted that a classmate with a prodigious memory also had protuberant eyes. When Gall in medical school learned that brain and behavior were related, he wondered if certain parts of the brain were responsible for certain abilities; if so, perhaps individuals with highly developed abilities had hypertrophy of appropriate brain regions. Perhaps, a faculty of memory was located in that portion of the brain just behind the eyes, explaining the combination of mental and anatomical aberrations in his childhood classmate.

Gall spent most of his adult life gathering cases of individuals with outstanding abilities (musical genius) or defects (homicidal maniac) associated with odd bumps on their skulls. He attributed most individual differences in skull shapes to changes in the underlying brain. In many instances, Gall actually obtained these skulls after death. Other individuals helped Gall in this burgeoning field of human endeavor, the most notable being Spurzheim, but the failure to find corroborative patterns began to erode the initial exuberance. Other people with prodigious memories did not have protuberant eyes. Phrenology became more and more popular as it

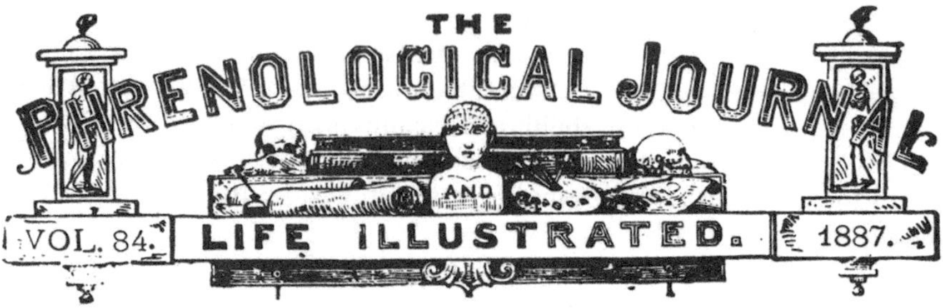

NUMBER 2.] *August,* 1887. [WHOLE NO. 584

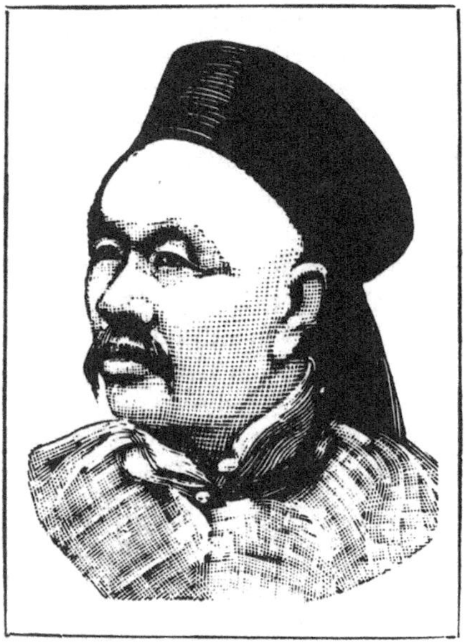

CHANG YEN HOON.

Figure 2: "The faculty we call Combativeness," says the phrenological report on the Chinese ambassador, "which lies at the foundation of assault and aggression, is not so strong in him as we sometimes find it, but the faculty we call Destructiveness is more strongly marked, and that gives severity, thoroughness, and the power to punish, and we think that is a Chinese peculiarity." And so on for 10 paragraphs.

became less and less scientific, until it gradually faded into an amusing parlor game.

Gall went way beyond his data, and his idea fell into disrepute. Today it seems droll to think that one can divide the personality into a specific number of discrete psychological faculties and to place each of these into a specific brain location. While it is true that a child's misshapen brain is accompanied by a misshapen skull, the concept that every slight bony prominence reflects an underlying brain prominence was too much to hope for. We also know today that interindividual personality differences of the kind examined by Gall are not generally reflected by gross changes in the size of brain regions. Nevertheless, Gall's basic ideas are the basis of modern neuropsychology; changes in brain anatomy and physiology correlate with changes in behavior. Animals raised in enriched environments will have a greater behavioral repertoire and thicker cerebral cortices than their littermates raised in impoverished environments (Rosenzweig and Bennett, 1972). Birds such as the owl, that use the sense of hearing for locating their prey at night, will have those portions of the brain dealing with sound analysis larger, and those portions concerned with visual analysis smaller than closely related birds such as the hawk, that hunt during the day using the visual sense.

The Bell-Magendie Law

At the same time phrenology was falling into disfavor, the experimental demonstration of localization of function in the nervous system began. Animal experimentation showed that cutting the anterior nerve root caused paralysis but no sensory loss, while section of the posterior root caused no motor change but the animal did not respond to painful stimulation. Similar surgical experiments with the cranial nerves showed the fifth to be predominantly sensory and the seventh to be predominantly motor.

These findings were uncovered at about the same time in the 1820's by both Sir Charles Bell in England and Francois Magendie in France. Even today we refer to a lesion of the seventh cranial nerve as "Bell's palsy." We say the discoveries were made by the two medical scientists at "about the same time," although an immediate vigorous debate arose concerning who did what first and who should get the most credit. Even today, historians differ over this issue.

Paul F. Cranefield has performed an important service by gathering all the original papers together in one volume entitled *The Way In and the Way Out*. Cranefield (1974) found that Bell's late review articles consistently aver that his earlier papers said more than they really did; Bell even misquotes himself within quotation marks. Cranefield feels that Magendie's superior experiments bring most of the credit for this momentous discovery to him. I agree that Magendie's original experiment was clearer than Bell's, and that Bell's personal behavior was reprehensible, yet, I think that most of the credit for bringing the importance of this discovery to the medical and scientific public belongs to Bell. Magendie's later experiments on peripheral nerves (rather than roots) failed to corroborate clear differentiation of function and he gave up this research pursuit; his physiology textbook does not even mention functional localization in the nervous system.

Regardless of who deserves what credit, the discovery of the differentiation of motor and sensory function in the peripheral nervous system ranks as the beginning of true scientific evaluation of localization of nervous function. It is eponymically remembered as the Law of Bell-Magendie.

The Whole Brain Counterreaction

The discrediting of phrenology saw a counterreaction to this school, which had so obviously overemphasized the relationship of mental faculties to localized brain regions. Most medical scientists in the middle of the nineteenth century held that psychological functions were a property of the entire brain. Simple sensory and motor functions, as shown by the Bell-Magendie Law, might be differentiated into different nerve fibers, but more complex functions—truly psychological functions—were related to the entire brain acting as a whole.

Animal experimentation seemed to corroborate this way of looking at brain function. Several experimentators had removed portions of the brain, especially cerebrum, in dogs and cats. The degree of postoperative deficit seemed more related to total volume than to location of tissue removed. A man named Goltz took his decorticate dog to international medical meetings to show how normal the animal looked at least to superficial observations.

The first unequivocal demonstration of localization of psychological function in man involved the demonstration of speech deficit following frontal lesions. Often, Broca is given credit for the popularization of this finding in the 1860's. Even within the field of aphasia, the degree of functional localization has shown marked swings of fashion. Broca held that the motor engrams responsible for muscular movements of tongue and throat that produce words were localized in the left third frontal convolution of the cerebral neocortex; a generation later, from further study of Broca's own initial case, Pierre Marie published a paper entitled, "The Third Frontal Convolution Has Nothing Particular To Do With Speech."

Failure to find a specific small brain lesion which would produce forgetfulness for a learned task was a great push toward the doctrine of non-localization. It appears that the search for a single, simple anatomical locus for each "memory engram" will forever fail. Lashley found that the ability of rats to run a familiar maze deteriorates proportionally to the volume of tissue removed, rather than its exact location. This finding reflected the less systematic observations from the previous century, and finds clinical correlation today in Alzheimer's disease where, in general, the degree of intellectual deterioration correlates with the amount of cortical atrophy.

Today

The two extremes are less marked today, but both have representatives. Localizationists seldom use the term "center" that was so popular just 20, or even 10 years ago. While one never sees the waking center or the various speech centers mentioned, the concept lives on with circuits or with neural programs, analogous to computer programs. The localizationists go beyond the data to name functions in the brain with the same overgeneralization from a single case which doomed the phrenologists.

The nonlocalizationist today accepts the functional differentiation of the two hemispheres but will go no further. His greatest strength is to recognize variation from one patient to another; his greatest weakness is an inherent vagueness.

In dealing with patients with organic brain disease, it is valuable to lean toward the localizationist position. Basically, this book overemphasizes cerebral localization of psychological function; its clinical strengths make this a valuable position to adopt.

Chapter 2

Lateralization of Psychological Function

INTRODUCTION

Each side of the brain controls the opposite side of the body. This holds true for sensory and motor function, with a few minor exceptions. The first portion of this chapter reviews thalamocortical input and corticoreticular output with the maximum brevity compatible with understanding. The second part of this chapter reviews the evidence for the separate psychological functions of each hemisphere.

MOTOR OUTPUT

Corticospinal Tract

It was long thought, and is still held as dogma by some, that the corticospinal tract is required for movement. If all corticospinal tract fibers were cut anywhere along their course through the brain, so the dogma goes, a complete and irreversible contralateral hemiplegia would invariably result. This theory, however, is not true.

The corticospinal tract originates in layers 5 and 6 (mainly layer 5) of the six-layered neocortex. Most fibers originate in the precentral gyrus, although a significant percentage arise from other portions of the neocortex.

The tract descends in the posterior portion of the posterior limb of the internal capsule, through the middle portion of the cerebral peduncle, to break up into separate smaller fascicles in the basis pontis, and then to reform into the medullary pyramid, a structure which gives the corticospinal tract its alternate name (Englander et al, 1975). The fibers cross at the lower end of the medulla, near the foramen magnum. These crossed fibers descend in the spinal cord along the lateral corticospinal tract to terminate on or near the anterior horn cell. A lesser number of uncrossed fibers descend along the ventral corticospinal tract.

Unfortunately for clinical pathological correlation, corticospinal fibers are seldom damaged alone. Large hemispheral lesions destroy the deep basal ganglia, as well as the cortical mantle. Even those small lacunar strokes which damage the corticospinal fibers in the posterior capsule also affect the ansa and fasciculus lenticularis as they exit the globus pallidus. Damage to the corticospinal tract in the basis pontis affects descending fibers from brain-stem nuclei, as well as cortical information on the way to the cerebellum. Similarly, hemisection of the spinal cord cuts reticulospinal fibers that are mixed with the lateral corticospinal tract. Only careful surgical removal of the neocortex destroys the pyramidal tract cells of origin, sparing deeper structures but not cortical input to them; damage to the pyramidal tract in the pyramids separates corticospinal from other motor influences. Damage in these areas causes contralateral transitory weakness, but not paralysis, and permanently increased contralateral tendon reflexes, absent abdominal reflexes, and a present Babinski sign (Meyer and Herndon, 1962; Bucy et al, 1964).

Basal Ganglia

The term basal ganglia refers to the masses of gray matter deep within the cerebral hemispheres. Originally, the term included the thalamus, but for functional reasons this has been separated, and the basal ganglia are presently defined to include the caudate nucleus, putamen, and globus pallidus with associated lesser nuclei, including the substantia nigra and the subthalamic nucleus of Luys. Caudate and putamen are probably functionally one nucleus broken into two fragments by the passage of the anterior limb of the internal capsule. Small clusters of myelinated fibers spread throughout the caudate and putamen give this structure a striated appearance and, hence, its alternate name, the corpus striatum. The putamen and globus pallidus, also called the pallidum, are shaped like a lens and are together termed the lenticular nucleus.

The major input to the basal ganglia arises from layer 5 of the cerebral neocortex. Greater input from frontal than from posterior lobe is reflected by the greater size of the head than the body and tail of the caudate nucleus. Major information flow through the basal ganglia proceeds from caudate to putamen, to globus pallidus.

Major output from the basal ganglia exits from the globus pallidus in two bundles, termed the fasciculus and ansa lenticularis. The fasciculus lenticularis passes through the posterior limb of the internal capsule, the ansa around it, to rejoin in the fields of Forel. Some fibers descend to the brain stem, while others form the thalamic fasciculus, which terminates in the ventral anterior and ventral lateral thalamic nuclei (predominantly the former). This region of the thalamus projects to layer 4 of the frontal neocortex, to affect corticospinal output and to complete a control loop—cortex to caudate, to putamen, to pallidum, to thalamus, back to cortex.

Interactions within the basal ganglia particularly involve substantia nigra. The dopaminergic nigrostriatal tract contains such small and diffuse fibers that this functionally important pathway was overlooked by classical neuroanatomy. Some fibers exiting the pallidum terminate in the subthalamic nucleus and affect movement by descending influences on brain-stem neurons, such as those in the red and facial nuclei and in the reticular formation. Lesions of the subthalamic nucleus result in uncontrollable, flailing movements of the contralateral limbs. The basal ganglia influences in the midbrain tegmentum probably affect the ipsilateral inferior olive via the central tegmental tract.

Cerebellum

The cerebellum relates to the contralateral cerebral cortex and basal ganglia (Asanuma and Hunsperger, 1975). Purkinje cell axons, always inhibitory, pass from cerebellar cortex to deep central cerebellar nuclei, especially the dentate nucleus. Dentate fibers exit via the superior cerebellar peduncle and cross the midline in the midbrain to the opposite red nucleus. Some synapse; others carry through the red nucleus to the ventral anterior and ventral lateral thalamic nuclei, predominantly the latter. This portion of the thalamus, as already mentioned, projects to layer 4 of the cerebral neocortex. Descending fibers from layer 5 complete a cerebellar control loop by descending through the anterior limb of the internal capsule and the cerebral peduncle to terminate in the basis pontis. Neurons in the basis pontis recross the midline to the granule cell layer of the cerebellum.

The basal ganglia and cerebellum interact in their effects on movement in the red nucleus and reticular formation of the brain stem, as well as through their interactions in the ventral anterior and lateral portions of the thalamus (Oka and Jinnai, 1978). Just as cerebral cortex influences contralateral cerebellum via corticopontine fibers, so the basal ganglia can influence the cerebellum via the descending central tegmental tract, which terminates on the ipsilateral inferior olive; olivocerebellar fibers then cross the midline and enter the cerebellum via the inferior cerebellar peduncle.

Other input to the cerebellum arises from the spinocerebellar tracts, which presumably carry feedback information concerning muscle contraction and position of limbs in space. Figure 1 summarizes these neuroanatomical connections.

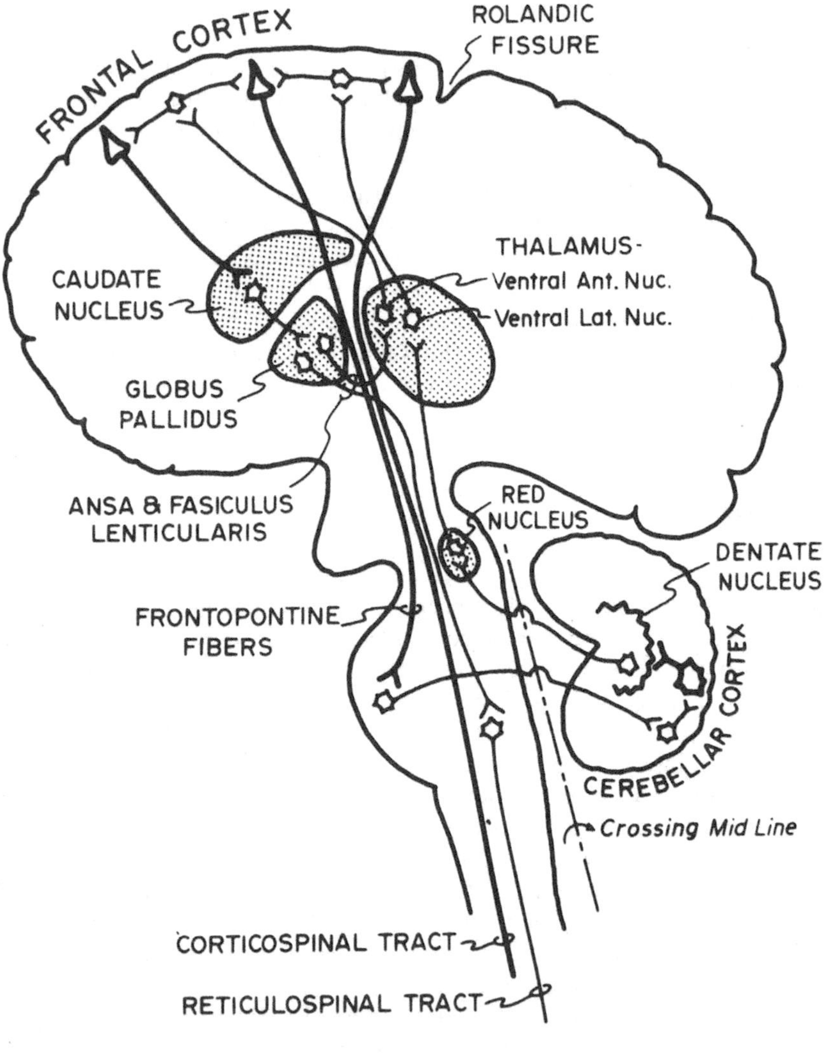

Figure 1: Cerebral cortex, basal ganglia, cerebellum, and reticular formation interact in the control of movement.

Motor Control

The neuroanatomy is well established; the exact neurophysiology of how the brain controls muscle contraction and movement remains somewhat sketchy. For the clinician who desires a somewhat oversimplified model which correlates with most observed clinical phenomena, the following one will do.

We begin by presuming that someone decides to move his arm, to pick up a pencil, for example. Somehow, this decision involves a change in neuronal activity in the cerebral neocortex. The exact correlation between the decision and the neuronal changes is so poorly understood that we don't even know how to phrase the question, but the details are irrelevant to this theory. The old concept described a direct cortical effect on the pyramidal tract, causing increased activity in appropriate anterior horn cells, muscle contraction of biceps, and arm movement. When the pyramidal tract was cut, the arm hung uselessly at the side. This old concept, bypassing cerebellum and basal ganglia, was oversimplified.

Actually, this cortical activity triggers a series of neuronal changes in basal ganglia analogous to a single command calling in a routine subprogram in a computer system. This subprogram has all the capabilities of making the movement, once the initial decision has been made. The movement subprogram changes pallidal output to thalamus, as well as to brain-stem descending tracts, such as the rubrospinal and reticulospinal tracts. The cerebellum enters the system because it contains information about pre-existing limb positions and muscle contractions. The movement program will be different if the arm is on the desk or behind the head, for example. The final milliseconds of the movement will involve impulses from visual cortex to cerebellum, and back to precentral gyrus and corticospinal tract—so-called eye-hand coordination. Figure 1 in the previous chapter illustrates this process.

The neocortex makes the decision. The basal ganglia contain the movement program. The cerebellum changes the movement program through its knowledge of present postural patterns. The corticospinal tract participates in the movement with other descending motor pathways and, because of its special endings near the anterior horn cells, makes the final corrective movements (especially of the fingers). Compare the way the brain controls movements with the way a pianist produces music. The muscles that actually move the limbs are like the piano wires that make the sounds. The anterior horn cells correspond to the hammers that fall upon the strings; different groups act together to produce different movements or different chords. The various descending tracts which transmit neuronal pattern changes in the brain to the anterior cells are like the complex mechanisms in the piano which transform movement of piano keys into the movement of the hammers on the wires. The keyboard is like the cerebellum/basal ganglia system. Perhaps, the interacting cerebellum and basal ganglia could be thought to correspond to the intermixed black and white keys. The influence of the motor neocortex on basal ganglia and cerebellum are like the fingers falling on the keys. The mystery of how a decision in the mind affects neocortical neurons is analogous to the mystery of how the brain and mind of the pianist can transform the concept of music into finger movements.

SENSORY INPUT

Vision

Considerable visual processing occurs within the retina. This information passes along the ganglion nerve fiber through the optic nerve, chiasm, and tract to synapse in the lateral geniculate body of the thalamus. Thalamocortical radiations project to layer 4 of the visual cortex in the occipital lobe (Weiskrantz, 1972).

Crossover within the optic chiasm is of such a nature as to allow one cerebral hemisphere to appreciate visual input from the opposite half of the environment. For species with laterally set eyes, such as the horse or pigeon, crossover is complete. Species with forward set eyes and depth perception, such as man, have crossover from the nasal retina, but ipsilateral projection from the temporal portion of the retina.

Hearing

The ossicles of the middle ear transduce sound waves into fluid waves within the endolymp of the cochlea. Specific hair cells trigger cochlear neurons when the fluid wave vibrates at specific frequencies. The cochlear nerve synapses in the various cochlear nuclei of the brain stem. This auditory information crosses the midline of the brain stem in the trapezoid body to ascend via the lateral lemniscus of the contralateral medial geniculate body of the thalamus. Thalamocortical radiations project to layer 4 of the auditory cortex in Heschl's gyrus of the temporal lobe. There is also a considerable projection ipsilaterally from cochlear nucleus via lateral lemniscus to ipsilateral medial geniculate body. The predominance of contralateral projection is shown by studies of bilateral auditory stimulation (dichotic listening), as reviewed in a subsequent section of this chapter.

Cutaneous Sensations

Fine-touch and position sensations proceed from the peripheral nerve up the ipsilateral posterior columns of the spinal cord, to the gracilis and cuneatus nuclei at the caudal end of the brain stem. This information crosses the midline at the sensory decussation and projects via the medial lemniscus to the ventral posterolateral (VPL) nucleus of the thalamus. Thalamocortical radiations project to layer 4 of the somesthetic cortex of the post-central gyrus in the parietal lobe—the so-called sensory strip or sensory homunculus.

Pain sensation from the body is conducted over peripheral nerves to the dorsal horn of the spinal cord. Traditionally, this was thought to synapse in the substantia gelatinosa, but recent anatomical studies show the connection between primary and secondary pain sensory neurons to take place more anteriorly in Rexed's lamina 5 and 6. This second cell projects via the lateral spinothalamic tract after crossing the midline in the spinal cord at the anterior white commissure. The spinothalamic tract terminates at the VPL, where pain sensation is integrated with other bodily sensations to project to the somatosensory cortex. Pain from the face proceeds by a homologous pathway from the trigeminal nerve to the spinal nucleus of the cranial nerve 5, crossing the midline to proceed rostrally as the quintothalamic tract and synapse in the ventral posterior medial (VPM) nucleus adjacent to the VPL. This information then projects to the face portion of the somatosensory gyrus. While this traditional pathway remains basically correct, recent research has shown that transmission through this system can be influenced by both peripheral and central (descending) input—the "gate" theory of pain (Wall, 1978). A comparison of the major senses is presented in Table 1.

Other Senses

Taste is also predominantly projected contralaterally, but details are not completely understood. It is not known if visceral sensation is to any degree lateralized. The sense of smell is handled by the brain in ways that are completely different than any other sense; it does not, for example, involve the thalamus. This is discussed in the next chapter.

In general, primary sensations are symmetrical. An exception described by Benton and his colleagues (1973, 1978) concerns the appreciation of the directional characteristics of a tactile stimulus across the palm. Right-handed subjects show superior directional judgement with the left hand, perhaps generalizing to the tactile sense the known superiority of the right hemisphere in visual spatial capabilities.

TABLE 1: Comparison of the Neuroanatomy of the Major Senses

Sense	*First Order Neuron*	*Second Order Neuron*	*Crossover*	*Prethalamic Tract*	*Third Order Neuron*	*Cortical Analyzer*
Sight	Bipolar cell of the retina	Ganglion cell of the retina	Optic chiasm	Optic tract	Lateral geniculate	Occipital cortex (area 17)
Hearing	Spiral ganglion cell	Cochlear nuclei	Trapezoid body	Lateral lemniscus	Medial geniculate	Heschl's gyrus (area 14)
Pain	Dorsal root ganglion cell	Dorsal horn of the spinal cord	Anterior white commissure	Spinothalamic tract	Ventrobasilar complex	Postcentral gyrus (area 3)
Position	Dorsal root ganglion cell	Gracilis and cuneatus nuclei	Sensory decussation	Medial lemniscus	Ventrobasilar complex	Postcentral gyrus (area 3)

HANDEDNESS

Approximately 90 percent of people write with their right hands. This is not only true of modern Western civilization, but of all societies that utilize writing. Reviews of ancient Egyptian murals show that approximately 90 percent of the individuals artistically represented were right-handed (Coren and Porac, 1977). Indirect evidence suggests that Neanderthal man and Homo erectus were also predominantly right-handed (Abler, 1976). The most ancient reference to handedness is recorded in Chapter 20 of the Book of Judges, describing a unit of 700 left-handed soldiers in an army of 26,000. This low percentage of left-handed people probably reflects another timeless principle: the disinclination of the soldier to volunteer for service in a special battalion. About 90 percent of people also favor the right leg for kicking, but a lesser majority, varying between 60 and 70 percent, favor the right eye for sighting (Porac and Green, 1976).

Why do the majority favor the use of the right hand? One of the oldest theories posits a survival advantage for individuals holding a weapon in the right hand and a shield in the left, over the heart. More fanciful suggestions relate to territoriality (Webster, 1977) or the use of the left hand to clean oneself after a bowel movement, keeping the right (or correct) hand clean for eating and for greeting (Sagan, 1977). The sinister connotations of the left remain today, as in the common exclamation, "I'm not going to see the movie starring that leftist no matter how good an actress she is." Froeschels (1961) thought handedness might be developed by a child solely from mimicry of his parents. We now know that some aspects of handedness must have a biological basis, because anatomical asymmetries are clearly present in the human brain.

In the general population of brains at autopsy, clear anatomical asymmetries exist. The left Sylvian fissure is longer, and the area on the upper surface of the left temporal lobe, medial to Heschl's gyrus is larger (Geschwind, 1978). Study of anatomical asymmetries in living humans using the CT scan reflect this asymmetry in right-handed individuals, but show greater variation in left handers. Similar anatomical asymmetries have been found in newborn infants and in some of the great apes. Cytoarchitectonic studies show greater cellular development in auditory- and speech-related regions of the left hemisphere (Galaburda et al, 1978). Neurochemical asymmetry in the normal human brain has been shown by Oke and co-workers (1978), who found a greater concentration of norepinephrine in the left than in the right pulvinar, that portion of the thalamus which connects with parietal cortex and Wernicke's area.

Virtually all right-handed people have speech represented in the left hemisphere. Evidence for this assertion occupies the remainder of this chapter.

Left-handed people seem to be more complex. Most of these individuals also have speech capabilities localized to the left hemisphere, but the percentage of this is lower. A few left-handed people are victims of perinatal distress, damaging the left hemisphere; the right develops speech because it is the only fully functional hemisphere and the individual becomes left handed because his right hand is not properly guided by the damaged left hemisphere. Statistical surveys show that left-handed people have greater perinatal morbidity, lower IQ, and more first born children than right handers because of this small subgroup of left handers with mild left brain damage (Bakan et al, 1973).

Left-handed people also show a greater bilaterality of function in many of the tests discussed in the rest of this chapter. Lesions of the dominant hemisphere do not produce as great a degree of aphasia as in right-handed people, and recovery is more rapid (Gloning, 1977). For these reasons, the remainder of this book refers to the right handed, unless otherwise specified. As an editorial shorthand, we will consider left hemisphere to be always speech related, knowing that we are excluding from analysis a small percentage of the general population.

LESIONS

Evidence for the lateralization of psychological function in man comes from three areas:

1) patients with lesions confined to one hemisphere;

2) normal subjects studied with speical techniques; and

3) a very few individuals who have their two hemispheres surgically separated for the treatment of epilepsy.

An adult with the sudden onset of complete left-hemisphere dysfunction, such as from a very large stroke, may or may not lose consciousness. If he does, it is for a brief period only. The patient has an obvious right hemiplegia with drooping of the right side of the mouth. He appears alert, but is almost speechless. He may just make a sound, like "uh," or he may say one or two simple words. He can shake his head to indicate yes or no, but has great difficulty understanding questions. Most patients can follow one simple command, like "raise your hand," but not complex ones like "touch your right eyelid with your left hand." The patient may take on a quizzical look when asked a question and many an examiner has been caught repeating questions louder and louder until he finds himself shouting at someone with perfectly normal hearing.

The adult with sudden dysfunction of the entire right hemisphere does not lose consciousness. He has a dense left hemiplegia; apparently the mirror image of the patient of the previous paragraph. Sometimes, the patient actually denies this hemiplegia, but this transient phenomenon passes quickly. The patient's speech, including reading and writing, seems completely normal, but he has a profound deficit of spatial abilities. He can not copy simple diagrams, nor can he identify locations on a map. His spouse frequently relates that he gets lost in very familiar surroundings. He has great difficulty recognizing faces and may develop the habit of not addressing a visitor, rather waiting for the visitor to speak first so that he can recognize the person by his voice.

We have been discussing complete and total destruction of one normal hemisphere with preservation of the other. Actually, of course, this never occurs. Occasionally, a very damaged and dysfunctional hemisphere is removed—a hemispherectomy—but the remaining hemisphere has been doing double work long before the surgery is performed. Some infarctions following sudden internal carotid artery occlusion are quite large, encompassing most of the hemisphere. But a lesion this large produces edema which may cause pressure on and dysfunction of the supposedly unaffected hemisphere.

In addition, the phenomenon generally given the term diaschisis complicates evaluation of function immediately after the infarction (Slater et al., 1977). When a source of synaptic input is removed, a transient period of depressed function will result. The most familiar form of this phenomenon is spinal shock; cut descending facilitatory synaptic bombardment and gamma loop reflexes will temporarily disappear. Similarly, when a portion of one hemisphere is removed, the homologous portion of the other hemisphere might have transiently depressed function, because of decreased synaptic bombardment through the cerebral commissures.

As diaschisis complicates the acute lesion, functional plasticity complicates the chronic. When a subject is tested months or years after a specific neurological deficit, the remaining portions of normal brain may have undergone significant reorganization. Functions of the destroyed tissue may have been taken over by the healthy tissue. This attempt at reorganization may be incomplete or even faulty, such as in the abnormal facial movements and tearing which can follow aberrant regrowth of cranial nerves.

Nevertheless, study of lesioned patients, especially stroke patients, remains the mainstay of clinical localization of function and separate chapters of this book are devoted to lesions of each hemisphere.

NORMAL SUBJECTS

A series of special techniques have attempted to demonstrate and evaluate lateralization in normal subjects. The first of these takes a cue from split-brain studies and communicates information directly to one hemisphere by flashing material to one visual field. The second presents different words simultaneously to both ears; results indicate that a word in the right ear is perceived better than the word spoken in the left ear. A third method measures blood flow to the two hemispheres during various types of mental operations. Several types of electroencephalographic changes show differential findings from the hemispheres during certain types of mental acts. Lastly, this section discusses pharmacological inactivation of a single hemisphere, by means of injection into a carotid artery.

Visual Stimulation Restricted to One Field

The basic hypothesis behind this type of research supposes that an object tachistoscopically flashed in one visual field will be perceived directly by the opposite hemisphere and subsequently be transferred to the other hemisphere via the corpus callosum. Suppose a normal right-handed subject is asked to press a button with his right hand whenever he sees a flash of light. If the light flashes in the right visual field (RVF), the perception and responses can be carried out in one hemisphere, from left visual cortex to the hand area in the left precentral gyrus and, then, via the corticospinal tract to the responding right hand. Light flashed in the LVF is carried to the right cortex (perhaps with a stopover in the left occipital cortex) and, hence, to the responding hand. Thus, when stimulation is in RVF, the reaction time should be shorter with right hand responding than with left. Similarly, LVF stimulation should be faster with the left hand responding. Actually, this has been shown many times, first by Poffenberger in 1912. The most careful measurements have shown that the reaction time delay is between two and three msec (Berlucchi et al., 1971). If two mirror points on two hemispheres were 10 centimeters apart and conduction velocity in the corpus callosum was 50 meters per second, the delay would calculate at two msec, for conduction time solely. Delay of passage at a synapse is about 0.5 msec.

The two hemispheres are apparently equal in this simple reaction time task. If a verbal response is required, rather than pressing a button, stimulation in RVF (direct communication to the left or speaking hemisphere) produces a faster response than LVF stimulation. Filbey and Gazzaniga (1969) found RVF to be about 30 msec faster than LVF. Amadeo and his co-workers found no such hemispheral delay, but the verbal response required of their subjects was a mere yes or no; suggesting perhaps that the right hemisphere can produce these words which are frequently little more than grunts associated with head shaking.

If one requires the subject to match a tachistoscopically presented visual image to a series of similar images, one finds faster performance when letters of the alphabet are flashed to RVF or photographs of faces are flashed to the LVF (Rizzolatti et al, 1971). The delays are approximately 15 msec. Learning an association between two symbols (one a single digit number) flashed to the same visual field is more easily accomplished in RVF than LVF (Dimond and Beaumont, 1974). Words flashed to RVF are more frequently recognized than when flashed to LVF (Hines, 1977). On the other hand, the LVF is superior in matching colors (Pennal, 1977) and in recognizing faces (Gilbert and Bakan, 1973). The latter phenomenon has been noted for many years, first by Wolff in 1933. Some had suggested that the phenomenon was in the face, not in the observer; perhaps the brain affected facial development asymmetrically, so that the right side of a person's face was more typcial of his entire face, while perhaps the left side of the face was more private or even "sinister." Using reversed photographs, Gilbert and Bakan (1973) showed conclusively that facial recognition was related to the visual field of the observer, not to any intrinsic facial characteristics.

Bilateral Auditory Stimulation

Auditory information presented to one ear is transmitted to both auditory cortices, even in the absence of intercerebral commissures. However, if two different words are simultaneously spoken to the two ears, subjects will most frequently say they heard the one in the right ear. This dichotic listening test, formalized with tape recording, shows that the right ear or left hemisphere is dominant for linguistic material (Kimura, 1967; Lowe et al., 1970). This right-ear superiority for language develops before the age of 5 (Berlin et al, 1973). Non-musicians recognize tunes better in the left ear, corroborating other evidence that musical appreciation is predominantly a right-hemisphere function (Bever and Chiarello, 1974). The situation is more complex for musicians, who apparently use analytic, left hemisphere functions in evaluation of musical material. The left ear or right hemisphere is also superior in judging the affective tone of recorded voices (Carmon and Nachson, 1973).

Electroencephalography

The most prominent characteristics of the resting, awake electroencephalogram is a regular 8 to 13 Hz rhythm, most prominent over the posterior half of the head. This is the alpha rhythm. While some have argued that this regular activity arises from a cranial structure other than the brain (Lippold and Novotny, 1970), careful studies in animals have unequivocally shown that this rhythm arises from the cerebral neocortex at the level of the large pyramidal cells (Lopes da Silva and Storm van Leeuwen, 1977).

In general, the alpha rhythm is best seen when the subject is awake, lying quietly with his eyes closed. The alpha is suppressed when the subject opens his eyes or if he drifts off to sleep. It is a commonplace observation in EEG laboratories that mental effort also suppresses alpha rhythm. If a subject lying quietly with his eyes closed is asked to perform an arithmetical problem in his head (a problem requiring some effort such as 27 times 7, not 3 plus 5), the alpha will disappear for a few seconds and then reappear just before he gives the answer. The electroencephalographer can stun the subject by requesting that he not give the answer; then, when the alpha returns, he can say, "Well, I see you have the answer." The subject gets the uncanny feeling that the EEG machine is reading his mind.

From these observations has come the working hypothesis that the alpha rhythm represents an "idling" state of the brain; the brain is alert and ready for information processing but is actually not involved in such processing at the present time. A further development of this hypothesis relates to asymmetric neuropsychological function. If one hemisphere became active, the alpha rhythm over this half of the scalp might drop in amplitude. According to existing concepts of hemisphere function, when the subject engaged in language or arithmetic tasks, alpha activity over the left half of the head would decrease more than on the right, and vice versa for a subject engaged in purely musical or spatial thinking.

In most normal right-handed people, the alpha rhythm is bilaterally symmetrical in frequency, but slightly greater in amplitude over the right hemisphere. This amplitude asymmetry is increased when subjects engage in language or in calculations, and is decreased or even reversed when subjects engage in tasks involving spatial or musical concepts (Doyle et al., 1974; Morgan et al., 1974; Bennett and Trinder, 1977; Hirshowitz et al., 1978). A negative report was complicated by the requirement that the subjects write their response to the mental task (Chartock et al., 1975). Alpha asymmetry is produced by subjects imagining visual forms or language, as well as performing preset tasks (Robbins and McAdam, 1974). Subjects who are not musicians have more alpha on the left when whistling a tune, more on the right when speaking the lyrics to the same tune, and little alpha asymmetry when singing the song (Davidson and Schwartz, 1977). The magnitude of the alpha asymmetry is related to the difficulty of the task, the rate at which it is performed, and the subject's age (Glass and Butler, 1977; McLeod and Peacock, 1977). Variations of alpha activity within the left hemisphere have been shown by Stigsby et al (1977); alpha suppression occurs more in the temporal lobe during an auditory memory test and more in occipital lobe during a visual reasoning test.

All the studies so far discussed have used various measures of alpha activity to show hemisphere specialization for psychological function. Other EEG measures also show hemispheral asymmetries. The potential which occurs after a specific stimulus is usually buried within ongoing activity, but averaging techniques allow a complex but reproducible picture of this evoked potential to emerge. Visually evoked potentials are usually of slightly greater amplitude over the right hemisphere (Rhodes et al., 1975). Left-hemisphere potentials, evoked by linguistic auditory stimuli are different from right; non-linguistic evoked potentials show no such asymmetry (Schucard et al., 1977). Slow negative potentials, probably related to the well studied contingent negative variation (Teece, 1971) are at a maximum over the left frontal region when the subject is speaking (McAdam and Whittaker, 1971; Grozinger et al., 1975).

The Wada Test

The Wada test is never performed in normal subjects, because it involves risk which can only be accepted when there is reasonable expectation of greater clinical benefit. Many subjects are psychologically normal without prior or subsequent evidence of organic mental disease, however, so this type of evaluation is discussed here.

The Wada test requires placement of a needle or catheter into the carotid artery, hence it is usually performed at the same time as cerebral angiography. After the angiogram is performed, a depressant drug, usually a barbiturate, is injected directly into the artery. The drug is carried to one hemisphere and "puts it to sleep." The subject is then examined presumably with only the other hemisphere active. Practically speaking, the examiner has only about a minute until the depressant drug travels through the heart going back through the circulation to the whole brain, making the subject too sleepy to continue. The angiogram must be checked to be sure that aberrant arterial development, such as both anterior cerebral arteries filling from the same carotid, does not deliver the depressant drug to both hemispheres. Vascular anatomy dictates that for most (but not all) people, only the anterior two-thirds of each hemisphere is depressed during the Wada test. The subject is asked to stretch both arms in front of him and count. If the right carotid is injected, the left arm falls, sometimes quite heavily, while the subject keeps counting; if asked to hold out the paralyzed arm, he usually replies something to the effect that it *is* held out. If the left carotid is injected, the right arm falls and the subject stops counting. He makes no effort to count but lies there quietly, looking blandly at the examiner who is urging him to continue counting. Occasionally, the left carotid injection produces immediate loss of consciousness with both arms falling limply and loss of head posture, closing of the eyes, and unarousability.

Other Studies in Normal Subjects

Electrical stimulation of language-related areas of the left hemisphere in psychologically normal subjects undergoing neurosurgical extirpation of epileptic brain tissue produces inability to name objects. Stimulation at the lateral portion of the precentral gyrus (the so-called face area) can produce speech arrest—inability to make any sound. Anterior to this region, in Broca's area, and in many regions of the left parietal and adjacent portion of the left temporal lobe, electrical stimulation produces a more specific anomia or inability to name. Shown a picture, the subject says, "That is a . . . , that is a . . . ," but can not come up with the word, later reporting an apparent mental block (Whittaker and Ojemann, 1978).

Several different experimental techniques have shown that blood flow increases to the left hemisphere when the subject speaks, reads, or calculates, while blood flow to the right hemisphere increases when the subject performs spatial pattern recognition problems (Carmon et al., 1972; Ingvar and Schwartz, 1974; Rosberg et al., 1975).

SURGICAL SEPARATION OF THE HEMISPHERES

Introduction

Despite a complete regimen of anticonvulsant drugs, some epileptic patients continue to suffer from frequent seizures. Of the many neurosurgical attempts to decrease the frequency of epileptic attacks, corpus callosal section has been attempted in a few cases. Van Wagennan performed partial callosal cutting in the 1930s, but had little success. More recently, the surgical approach has been expanded to include complete section of the corpus callosum as well as the anterior and hippocampal commissures. In many cases, this operation decreases the number and the severity of epileptic seizures. The procedure has been adapted for infants and children (Lussenhop et al., 1970). Special psychological study of these unique individuals has expanded our knowledge of hemisphere specialization (Dimond, 1972; Gazzaniga, 1970).

The surgical approach is through a right frontoparietal craniotomy. The right hemisphere is gently retracted laterally and the corpus callosum is exposed. The callosal commissure is divided slightly to the right of the midline to avoid midline blood vessels. The fornices are cut near the foramen of Monro and this section is continued anteriorly to include the anterior commissure. When present, the thalamic massa intermedia is also divided.

The immediate post-operative period demonstrates transient neurological deficits. For several hours after regaining consciousness, hypotonia is present—more markedly in the left arm than the right. Forced grasping and Babinski signs are present bilaterally immediately after surgery, with the right abnormality usually disappearing before the left. The immediate post-operative neurological status of commissurectomy patients is described by Gazzaniga, Bogen, and Sperry (1967):

> All patients except one . . . showed good control of movements of the right arm and leg within a few hours after surgery. At the same time all patients showed in some degree left-sided apraxia to verbal commands. For example, spoken commands such as "Raise your left arm," "move your left foot," "Make a fist with your left hand," could not be carried out.

Most studies have evaluated these patients months to years after commissurotomy, long after these transient neurological abnormalities have disappeared.

The most carefully studied individuals are the patients of Bogen and Vogel in Los Angeles. Clinical and testing information concerning the most frequently studied cases is summarized in Table 2. Our knowledge gained from these six subjects is amplified by reports of single unusual cases, such as a patient with chronic focal brain injury (Nebes and Sperry, 1971), and a patient studied with intraoperative electroencephalography (Torres and French, 1973). Goldstein and Joynt (1969) reevaluated a case operated upon by Van Wagennan and found that few changes in psychological function had occurred during the passage of 27 years. Patients with partial callosal section show very little of the extensive syndrome which usually follows complete cutting of interhemispheric connections. Section of the posterior portion of the corpus callosum produces a few changes in visual testing only (Gazzaniga and Freedman, 1973), while anterior callosal section causes only very slight changes in bimanual fine motor skills (Gordon et al., 1971; Preiloski, 1972).

In most tests, the subject is seated before a screen and told to fix his gaze at a certain point. Images flashed more than 10 degrees to the right of this fixation point are communicated only to the left hemisphere. The subject can describe these images. Images flashed more than 10 degrees to the left of the fixation point are perceived only by the right hemisphere. These cannot be

TABLE 2: Variation in Test Results in Six Commissurized Individuals

				Letter Recognition				*Figural Unification*	
				Left Hemisphere		*Right Hemisphere*			
Patient	*Sex*	*Age at Injury*	*Age at Operation*	*Pointing*	*Stating*	*Pointing*	*Stating*	*Left Hemisphere*	*Right Hemisphere*
AA	M	Birth	13	97%	91%	47%	22%	45%	85%
CC	M	Birth	13	91	100	38	22	30	70
NG	F	Birth	20	88	94	44	16	35	75
LB	M	Birth	13	97	94	53	38	85	100
NW	F	3	36	97	72	41	0	40	85
RY	M	3	43	97	97	25	19	35	80

Note the bilaterality of function in LB. The letter recognition test of Teng and Sperry (1973) involves the recognition of letters flashed to one visual field and their identification by pointing (easier) or verbal report. The figural unification of Nebes (1973) requires the subject (or his hemisphere) to identify a puzzle piece from its tactual characteristics explored with one hand.

described verbally, but the patient can, with his left hand, point at the presented image in a series of pictures or can, by palpation, select a three dimensional representation of the image blindfolded. Some studies have used electrophysiologic recording of eye movements to eliminate a momentary turning of the eyes toward the flashed image as a cause of visual communication to both hemispheres.

Perception

It seems that tactile sensation from the hand is transmitted predominantly to the contralateral hemisphere. Objects in the left hand cannot be verbally identified, but can be pointed out, even after a delay, thus indicating that stereognostic information is transmitted to the right hemisphere and can be remembered. The amount of somatosensory information transmitted to the ipsilateral hemisphere increases with the passage of time following commissurotomy. In the early post-operative period, blindfolded subjects can point to stimulated body areas only with the hand ipsilateral to the stimulation. Indication of points across the midline can be accomplished only on the face and tongue. Retesting after a period of years, however, has shown that either hand can point to the site of stimulation anywhere on the body, but the contralateral hand (or ipsilateral hemisphere) is unable to demonstrate the direction in which a stylus is drawn across a body surface (Norrsell, 1973).

In all patients studied, except L.B., the subject with marked bilaterality of psychological function, olfactory stimulation was strictly unilateral. With the right nostril occluded by digital pressure, subjects can verbally identify odors. Occlusion of the left nostril, but not the right, however, prevents accurate verbal description of odors. The individual can indicate with his left hand an object associated with the odor; for example, he points at a plastic toy fish after being presented with a fishy odor, or he indicates a small coffee cup after smelling coffee. These results indicate that olfactory information is transmitted to the ipsilateral hemisphere. The speaking hemisphere can describe the odor; the right hemisphere can indicate an object generally associated with the odorous substance (Gordon and Sperry, 1969).

Visual information from the contralateral field is delivered via optic tract, lateral genticulate body, and geniculocalcarine radiations to each hemisphere in an identical manner. This primary visual information is processed differently, however, in the two hemispheres. The earliest studies noted that complex pictures flashed to the RVF could be accurately described, while those presented to the LVF were described only as a flash of light. Later evaluation showed that some patients could not only describe a pinpoint light source in the LVF, but could also indicate by hand movements or by speech the direction of movement of this point of light. The detailed visual function studies of Trevarthen and Sperry (1973) have shown that commissurotomized patients have some ability to perform analyses requiring comparison of visual stimuli in the LVF with those in the RVF. For example, the subject notes that he sees a "twisting movement" when one point of light moves upward in one visual field and another moves downward in the other visual field. The subject can indicate the midpoint of an imaginary line connecting a point in one field with a point in the other field. Subcortical areas, probably including the superior colliculi, presumably have this ability to organize information from peripheral vision. This analysis is communicated to the left hemisphere where it can be translated into verbal descriptive output.

Motor Control

In general, each hemisphere has best control over the contralateral hand, but on certain occasions one hemisphere can control both hands. Axial and facial musculature can be controlled by either hemisphere. For example, the

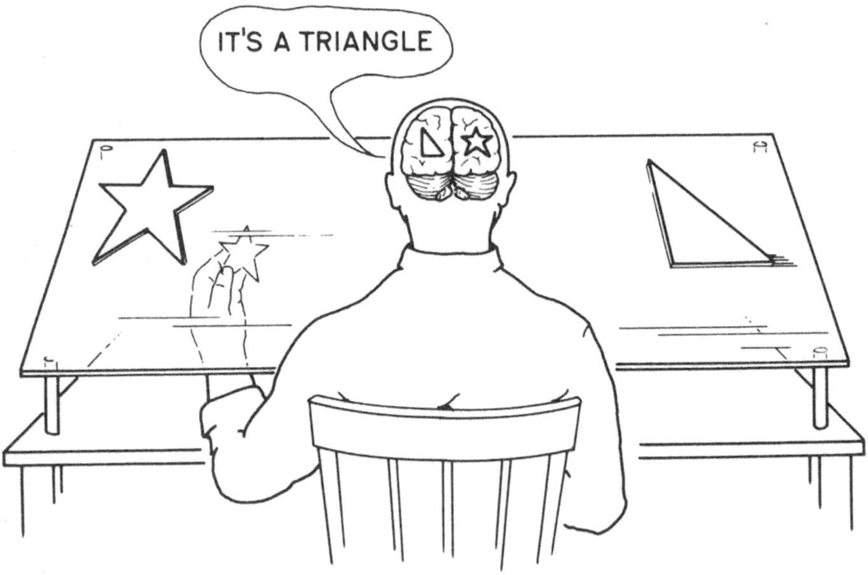

Figure 2: Cutting the corpus callosum produces poor communication between the hemispheres. "Find with your left hand what you saw flashed on the screen." The left hand gropes for the star. "Now what do you have?" The speaking hemisphere saw the triangle and assumes that is what is in the hand. From a drawing by Timothy F. Nolan, M.D.

written word *smile* flashed to the RVF causes the subject to perform this written command. Apparently then, the left hemisphere has total control of the motor mechanisms which produce the act of smiling. The written word *smile* flashed to the LVF causes no action, but the picture of a smiling mouth causes the subject to smile, a motor act presumably initiated in this case by the right hemisphere. While this hemisphere has only limited ability to understand written commands, it very regularly initiates acts that are demonstrated by pictures. Either hemisphere can initiate acts involving facial or axial musculature or proximal movements of either arm, but there is less control over ipsilateral finger movements. Pictures of complex finger postures flashed to either visual field can be reproduced perfectly by the hand ipsilateral to the field (contralateral to the hemisphere receiving the visual information and initiating movements), but the other hand has some difficulty. This was referred to by Gazzaniga and his co-workers (1967) as apraxia. In general, right hemisphere control over the right hand is poorer than left hemisphere control over the left hand.

Evidence suggests that the two hemispheres exert alternating control over the motor mechanisms of the central nervous system which initiate and guide muscular movements. For example, introduction of a malodorous vapor into the right nostril produces a disgruntled facial expression and a vocal emittance of dissatisfaction such as "yuk," followed by a smile and a verbal statement about the odor such as, "Boy, that was a bad one." The right hemisphere produced the initial facial expression, the left subsequent speech. The right hemisphere controlled respiratory musculature to produce the initial grunt, then the left assumed control to produce the verbal description. The left hemisphere was not responding directly to the odor, of course, which it had not experienced, but rather was responding to the facial expression and grunt produced by the right hemisphere. This cross-cue permits the right hemisphere, which experiences the odor, to communicate an aspect of the odor—its unpleasantness—to the speaking hemisphere.

Another example of alternation of motor control derives from cross-cueing of visual images. An object is flashed to the LVF and recognized by the right hemisphere. If the subject is asked to name the object, his left hemisphere assumes control over the speech musculature and the patient speaks words indicating that he saw no identifiable object. If the person is then asked to select the object from a group, he may point to it with his left hand and then name it. The right hemisphere controls the pointing, the left hemisphere sees the indicated object and then, through control of the speech musculature, speaks its name. The actual act of pointing is not necessary; the fixation of eyes upon the object is all that is needed. The right hemisphere produces this ocular fixation and the speaking hemisphere merely observes the object and names it. After reviewing evidence for alternation of motor control, Nebes (1974) concluded:

> These results point to a response hierarchy in terms of competing responses programmed by the two hemispheres, with the hemisphere whose speciality the task demands gaining access to the motor system. This decision between the two hemispheres' claim to the response apparatus might well be a result of cortical influences balancing out at the brainstem level.

Under certain conditions, the right hemisphere can direct left hand and finger movements while the left hemisphere controls the right hand. This is shown by experiments in which the right hand presses one or another button if a red or green color appears in the RVF, while the left hand performs a similar discrimination test of light and dark stimuli appearing in the LVF. Normal subjects are markedly slowed by this double discrimination, but commissurotomy patients can perform both discriminations as rapidly as either alone (Gazzaniga and Sperry, 1966). Presumably, each hemisphere solves its own discrimination problem and controls the contralateral hand without reference to the activities of the other hemisphere. Tapping with either index finger can be performed by the commissurotomized subject at the same rate as the normal person, but attempts to tap both fingers results in a slower tapping rate (Kreuter et al., 1972). In one subject, simultaneous performance of verbal tasks disrupted tapping with the right index finger only, demonstrating that each hemisphere was controlling the contralateral index finger.

Psychological Function

Standard psychological testing of the commissurized person reveals little effect of this rather extensive surgery. There are no changes in measured temperament or intelligence. Relatives report, however, that these subjects frequently forget telephone messages and appointments, and some standard tests such as the Wechsler Memory Scale reveal a moderate deficit of short-term memory (Zaidel and Sperry, 1974). More extensive interviewing sometimes reveals that the patient's two hands may at times seem to work at cross purpose. One subject revealed an occasion when he tried to take his trousers off with his right hand but pull them on with his left. Another patient's wife described an evening when her husband picked up a newspaper with his right hand, abruptly put it down with his left, and had to pick it up again with his right. Occasionally during testing, a subject remarks that his left hand "acts on its own" or "seems to have a mind of its own."

The left hemisphere has the complete verbal and calculating abilities of a normal person. Every commissurotomized subject can name and describe in detail images in the RVF. With the right hand, these patients can write from dictation or write descriptions of pictures flashed in the RVF and of objects felt out of sight by the right hand. When these same stimuli are presented to the LVF, no written response is possible. Several months post-operatively, two of the patients were able to write with their left hands, mostly controlled from the proximal shoulder and elbow joints, not the fingers. This was still being controlled by the left hemisphere, however, since they still could not write words presented to the LVF (Gazzaniga and Sperry, 1967). Calculation problems presented to the RVF or the right hand were performed the same before as after commissurotomy. With numbers presented by feeling with the left hand, the right hemisphere demonstrated a limited ability to add single digits but was unable to subtract or multiply. If a set of from one to four wooden pegs is presented to the patient's left hand, out of view and in random order, the patient can readily pick out blocks of requested numerical value. The subjects are usually unable to subtract the number of pegs in one block from those in another, or to double or triple the number of pegs.

Though deficient in verbal and calculating abilities, the right hemisphere surpasses the left in tasks involving spatial form, including the recognition of faces. The interpretation of spatial organization is better performed by the right hemisphere. While the left hand can correctly reassemble complex patterns and puzzles, the right hand can only reproduce the simplest test, and often the left hand spontaneously jerks up and tries to help the awkward right hand. Failure ensues when both hands are allowed to work "together," since the right hand undoes any constructive work accomplished by the left hand.

Nebes (1973) studied the ability of commissurotomized patients to interpret arrays of dots. Regardless of whether the right or left hand was used in answering (only a finger twitch was required), the number of patterns correctly interpreted was always higher when presented to the LVF than the RVF. A normal control group showed no difference between the two fields. Milner and Taylor (1972) tested spatial memory abilities of the right hemisphere. A simple pattern or object was placed out of sight in one hand for 10 seconds. After varying delay periods, the subject was then asked to retrieve it from a set of four shapes, still out of sight. Even with a zero delay, the left hemisphere has difficulty with this type of task. For periods of two minutes or longer, however, the right hemisphere can remember the shape and correctly retrieve it. Levy and his colleagues (1972) projected a chimera (one picture composed of two different halves) to the visual midline of commissurotomized patients, then with a group of normal pictures in free view before them, directed them to point to the pictures they had seen. In such cases, the picture indicated was always that one whose half had appeared in the LVF. When asked to describe the face or object seen, subjects described the face in the RVF. This indicated that if a language related answer is required, the left hemisphere controls behavior. With verbal interaction eliminated, the image in the right hemisphere dictates the motor response. At no time did any of the patients indicate that they had seen two different pictures.

Two representative studies indicating verbal superiority of left and spatial superiority of right hemisphere are summarized in Table 2.

Two Minds in Every Head?

The results cited seem to show that two separate mental organizations exist in each commissurotomized individual. Investigators working with these patients were forced to postulate the existence of two separate thinking apparati when they attempted to describe their results. The total person says he saw nothing in his left visual field, but his left hand selects the object; the left or speaking hemisphere saw nothing, but the right can retrieve the object or one related to it. The "two minds" concept followed from the practical problem of referring to the perception and information processing technique of each hemisphere. Some early commentators considered the left hemisphere to be truly human and the right to be only a sensorimotor amalgam, little different from the right hemisphere of a chimpanzee or perhaps even a dog or cat. But further examination of the abilities of the so-called minor hemisphere revealed striking human qualities. It can associate the odor of coffee with a cup and saucer, or hydrogen sulfide with the plastic model of a fried egg; it can count and can recognize simple words. Its performance in some areas, such as the recognition of faces is clearly superior to the ability of the left "mind." Every author who has reviewed this problem recently has concluded that commissurotomized subjects contain two mental organizations. Each organization can, by special means, receive information not communicated to the other. Each can signal to the outside world the conclusions reached by its own thought process.

Most workers have concluded that in normal people, just as in these commissurotomized epileptic patients, two separate minds exist in each individual. Two personalities exist in all men, they say, commissurotomy merely uncovers and permits analysis of what is already present. Pucetti (1973) deduces from purely logical considerations that two personalities exist in every head; if they did not, he says, then the operation of commissurotomy would create two personalities from one. He feels that it is necessary to assume two personalities in every head, communicating and cooperating through the corpus callosum and other commissures:

> How can commissurotomy *create* two minds or persons if there

TABLE 3: Comparison of the Two Mental Organizations Present in Each Commissurotomized Patient

Anatomical Correspondence	*Left Hemisphere*	*Right Hemisphere*
Motor control	All but fingers of left hand	All but fingers of right hand
Speech abilities	Those of a "normal person"	Understands much speech, reads a few words, but can not speak or write
Calculating abilities	Those of a "normal person"	Very limited
Spatial abilities	Extremely limited	Apparently those of a "normal person"
Facial recognition	Extremely poor	Abilities of a "normal person"
Associative ability	Those of a "normal person"	A very high level

> was just one before? Which mind, the left-based one or the right-based one is brand new?

Careful application of the theory of psychophysical parallelism reviewed in the previous chapter permits an alternative, more logical explanation. Before the corpus callosum is sectioned, the brain is a single functional neural unit, producing (or more properly stated, corresponding to) a single mental experience. After the surgical section, two separate neural amalgams produce two apparent mental entities.

Chapter 3

The Limbic System

THE CONCEPT OF THE LIMBIC SYSTEM

A limbus is a rim or margin. In 1878, Broca suggested the term "limbic lobe" for those anatomical structures that encircle the third ventricle and the sagittally sectioned corpus callosum. This portion of the brain was thought to be functionally restricted to the perception of the sense of smell. In 1937, Papez reviewed clinical evidence suggesting that these medial structures and their connections were involved in emotion. MacLean (1949, 1952) proposed that these anatomical regions might together form a functional unit; he introduced the term "limbic system." The last two decades have seen a better definition of the anatomical interrelationships of structures within this system and an expansion of its borders to include parts of midbrain, thalamus, and neocortex. Some neuroanatomical authorities still resist the concept of a limbic system; for example, Brodal (1969) includes definite olfactory structures within the rhinencephalon and distributes other portions to the traditional cortico-thalamic-reticular system, doubting the existence of a limbic system as a functional entity. Livingston and Escobar (1971) argue that the anatomical expansion of this system beyond medial brain structures confuses the original limbic concept of Broca; they propose using the term limbic system to refer to the margin or edge which encircles the undersurface of the brain, as it is viewed following removal of brainstem and cerebellum.

Regardless of historical arguments and disagreements, evidence continues to accumulate supporting the view that these brain regions are related to emotion and especially to memory. This does not mean that other brain areas are not important in emotion and memory, since they are, nor does it mean that limbic areas do not interact with other systems such as the somatosensory system, for they do; but it does seem likely that this limbic system has some degree of functional autonomy. This chapter reviews the anatomical components of the limbic system, their connections, and the results of their destruction in man.

OLFACTION

The molecular mechanism by which odorous substances change the firing rates of fibers in the olfactory nerves remains unknown. The peripheral connections of these nerves are well established, but their centripetal projections disappear within the limbic system.

The olfactory nerve passes through the cribiform plate to the olfactory bulb. The extensive information processing which occurs in the bulb involves dendordendritic synapses (Shepherd, 1972). The mitral cells of the olfactory bulb have axons which project down the olfactory tract. Some of these synapse on neurons which are located all along the tract; these neurons are termed the anterior olfactory nucleus. The fibers of the olfactory tract divide to form the medial and lateral olfactory stria; a few fibers pass directly to the gray between these two stria, the anterior perforated substance—so named for the many small blood vessels which penetrate it. In animals with a well developed sense of smell, this region is much larger and is called the olfactory tubercle. The medial olfactory stria end in the septal nuclei and the parolfactory and subcallosal gyri. The lateral olfactory stria go to amygdala and overlying hippocampal gyrus—sometimes called parahippocampal gyrus to emphasize its separateness from pes hippocampus or hippocampus major. In macrosomatic mammals, this structure obtains a large size and is termed the piriform lobe.

The spherical mass of gray matter termed the amygdala lies anterior and just medial to the most rostral extent of the hippocampal gyrus. Various authors divide the amygdala of different species into several nuclei; in man, the amygdala contains two interconnected nuclei. The corticomedial nucleus receives fibers from the lateral olfactory stria and sends fibers via the stria terminalis in a great arc alongside the body and tail of the caudate nucleus to the ipsilateral preoptic and parolfactory areas, and through the anterior commissure to these same regions in the opposite hemisphere, as well as to the cortico-medial portions of the opposite amygdala. The basolateral portion of the amygdala is much larger than the corticomedial portion in man, in contradistinction to the opposite situation in mammals with a highly developed sense of smell, such as the dog.

The implanted brain electrode studies of Halgren and co-workers (1977) prove unequivocally that basolateral amygdala in man is not directly related to olfaction. This region of the amygdala receives input from the overlying hippocampal cortex and from the dorsomedial thalamic nucleus (Nauta,

1962); output is to the neocortex on the undersurface of the temporal lobe, to the preoptic area and hypothalamus, through the anterior commissure to the opposite basolateral amygdala, and via the roundabout route of the stria terminalis indirectly to these same areas. The basolateral amygdala also sends fibers via the uncinate fasciculus to the orbital and medial frontal cortex, and via the cingulum to cingulate cortex.

The medial olfactory related structures of septal nuclei and subcallosal and parolfactory gyri receive input from medial olfactory stria and median forebrain bundle. This latter tract interconnects these regions with orbito-frontal cortex, with preoptic and hypothalamic regions, and with certain midbrain nuclei. The septal nuclei, usually referred to simply as the septum (though only a few nerve cells are located within the septum pellucidum), also receive input from the hippocampus via precommissural fibers of the fornix (Siegel et al., 1975). Efferent fibers from the septum travel via the fornix to terminate in the hippocampal complex (Raisman et al., 1965).

HIPPOCAMPAL FORMATION

The hippocampal complex consists of the dentate gyrus, Ammon's horn or the pes hippocampus, the various subicular areas, and the overlying hippocampal cortex. The latter forms both an anatomic and a phylogenetic junction between the adjacent six-layered neocortex of the fusiform and inferior temporal gyri, and the more primitive subicular areas deep to Ammon's horn. The dentate gyrus and Ammon's horn are three-layered structures related to each other like two interlocking horseshoes. Input to the hippocampal gyrus comes from adjacent cortical areas, prefrontal cortex, basolateral amygdala, septum, and probably many other portions of the brain (Leichnetz and Astruc, 1975). The predominant flow of information within the hippocampal complex is from the hippocampal gyrus to dentate gyrus, to Ammon's horn and the subiculum. Pyramidal neurons of the hippocampal gyrus synapse in the molecular layer of the dentate gyrus; neurons within the middle layer of this gyrus, in turn, synapse on the long dendritic processes of Ammon's horn. The pyramidal cells of Ammon's horn send their axons into the great outflow system of the hippocampal complex—the fornix. These axons draw together into the body of the fornix which passes along the most medial and superior portion of the lateral ventricle. Some fibers pass rostral to the anterior commissure to synapse in the septum, the preoptic area, and the anterior hypothalamus. Those fibers caudal to the anterior commissure descend in the column of the fornix to synapse in the posterior hypothalamus, predominantly in the mammillary body. A few subicular axons project directly to the anterior thalamic nucleus, bypassing the larger pathway through the mammillary body

(Meibach and Siegel, 1977). Some fibers in the fornix cross the midline via the hippocampal commissure to the opposite hippocampal complex.

HYPOTHALAMUS

The hypothalamus is continuous anteriorly with the preoptic area, and posteriorly with the gray masses of the central midbrain. It has been divided into various nuclei and areas by several anatomists, but only a few nuclei stand out as distinctive cell masses. The periventricular and centromedial nuclei send their axons to the pars nervosa of the pituitary gland, where they discharge the peptide hormones oxytocin and antidiuretic hormone. The periventricular nucleus receives input from surrounding hypothalamic regions, via the median forebrain bundle from medial frontal and orbital cortex, and from brain stem structures. The centromedial nucleus receives

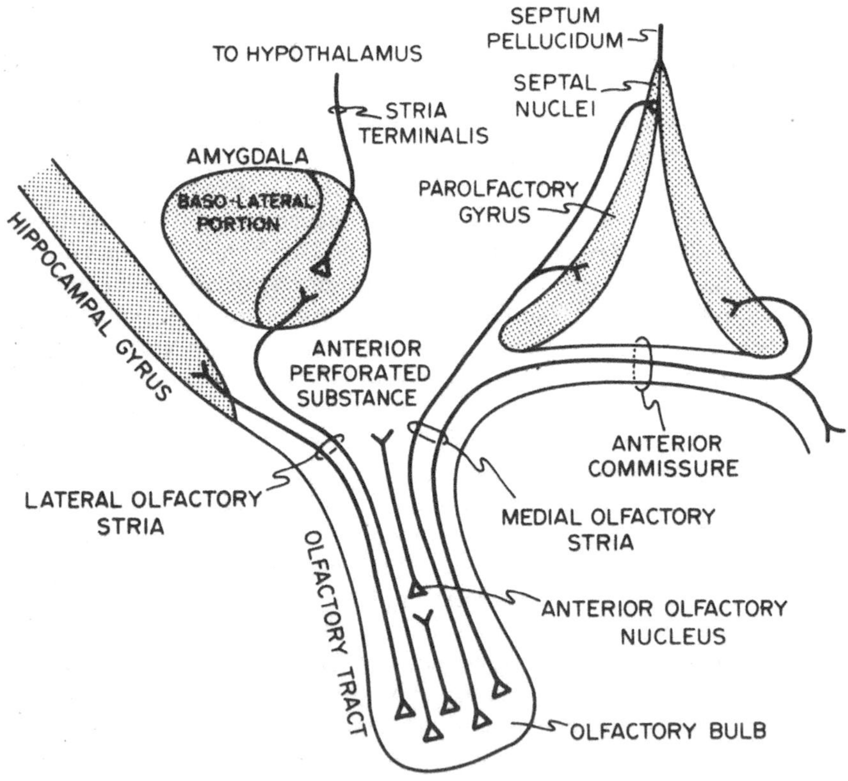

Figure 1: The limbic system receives and processes olfactory information.

input from surrounding hypothalamic and preoptic regions and from the amygdala via the stria terminalis. The mammillary body has major input from the hippocampus via the fornix and communicates to the anterior nucleus of the thalamus via the mammillothalamic tract. Nuclei of the mammillary bodies interact via the mammillary peduncle with brain stem structures, including the interpeduncular area, ventral tegmental gray, and the fasciculus solitarius. The anterior hypothalamic area receives input from surrounding regions, including the preoptic area and septum, and probably from rostral cortical regions, including parolfactory and subcallosal gyri and orbital gyri. The stria medullaris connects the anterior hypothalamus and preoptic area with the ipsilateral habenuala and, via the habenular commissure, with the contralateral habenula (Kataoka et al, 1977). The median forebrain bundle courses through the lateral hypothalamic area. The posterior hypothalamus has major connections with the hippocampus via the fornix and with adjacent areas caudally in the midbrain, including the periaqueductal gray region.

A major aspect of hypothalamic informational input involves intrinsic chemoreceptors. Portions of the medial hypothalamus are separated from third ventricular fluid by an unusual type of ventricular lining, and chemicals secreted into the third ventricle by other neural elements may effect neuronal activity in the median eminence and arcuate nuclei, as well as subsequently other adjacent hypothalamic and hypophyseal elements (Weindl, 1973).

A major outflow of the entire hypothalamus is the dorsal longitudinal fasciculus, originating in anterior, lateral, and posterior hypothalamic areas, and coursing caudally in the dorsal brainstem to synapse ipsilaterally in autonomically related areas, including the nucleus of Edinger-Westphal, the salivatory nuclei, the dorsal tegmental nucleus, and the facial nucleus where it may influence emotional facial expression.

The other major functional efferent from the hypothalamus is its effect on the anterior pituitary gland. In addition to the three sex hormones, luteinizing hormone, follicle stimulating hormone, and prolactin, the anterior pituitary gland secretes growth hormone, thyroid stimulating hormone (TSH), which stimulates the synthesis and secretion of thyroxine, and adrenocortical stimulating hormone (ACTH), which regulates the secretion of adrenal glucocorticoids. The rate of synthesis and release of all these polypeptide hormones is regulated by small peptides synthesized in the hypothalamus, mainly in the median eminence, and carried to the anterior pituitary by a vascular portal system. The amino acid sequences of some of these peptides have been discovered and have been synthesized for clinical research. Five of the six hormones of the anterior pituitary are predominantly under the control of releasing factors, while prolactin is inhibited by the hypothalamic portal system. Separation of anterior pituitary from hypothalamic control as by stalk section causes a depression of most hormones, especially TSH and the gonadotropins, but prolactin becomes elevated and nonpregnant lactation can result. This can also occur following certain types of hypothalamic damage or by inhibition of prolactin inhibitory factor by certain drugs, such as the phenothiazines. A patient with decreased pituitary function associated with elevated prolactin secretion has a greater likelihood of harboring a hypothalamic lesion than a patient with complete panhypopituitarism.

Recent advances in the understanding of growth-hormone control are beginning to have clinical relevance. Growth hormone is secreted by the adenohypophysis in bursts following stress, exercise, fever, hypoglycemia, and the onset of sleep. This is presumably due to changes over short time periods in the secretion of growth hormone releasing factor (GRF) by neuronal processes in the median eminence, with subsequent transfer down the portal system to pituitary cells. In experimental animals, electrical stimulation of the arcuate or ventromedial nuclei or (according to some investigators) of the amygdala causes a marked and prompt elevation of serum growth hormone. In man, these stimulatory influences contain a dopaminergic component, since oral levodopa, the precursor of dopamine, produces a definite rise of growth hormone in Parkinsonian patients as well as normal subjects. There seem to be some species differences, since in rats levodopa does not cause growth hormone secretion (Muller, 1973). The first hour of sleep produces a very marked rise of serum growth hormone. This could be due to influences of the raphe nuclei, related to sleep onset in cats and possibly in man, upon the hypothalamus via serotonergic fibers of the median forebrain bundle.

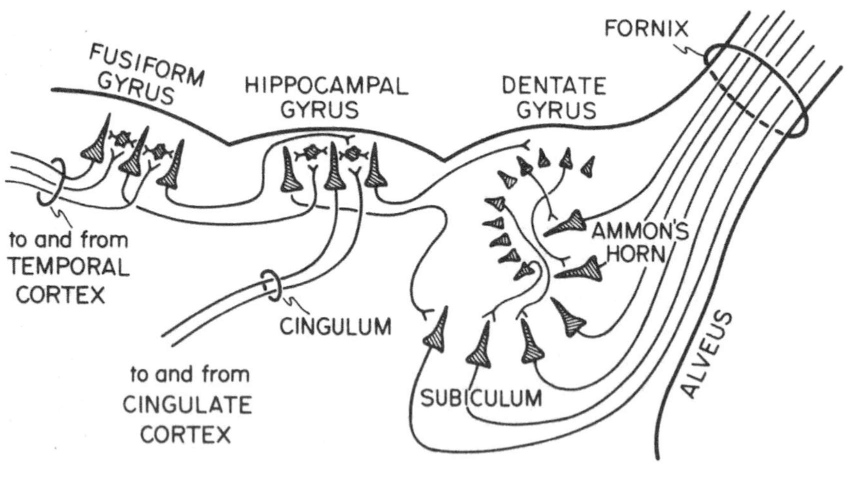

Figure 2: Limbic neocortex provides the major input to the hippocampal system; the predominant outflow is via the fornix.

The anterior hypothalamus has, in general, an inhibiting influence upon GRF activity, since destruction of this area causes a rise in total 24-hour values of growth hormone. Hypoglycemia is a potent stimulus of growth-hormone release. This is presumably due to receptors within the hypothalamus, since isolated hypothalamic-pituitary islands still show a growth-hormone response to hypoglycemia. Growth-hormone physiology is of value in studying incidents of hyposecretion producing growth retardation in children, and incidents of hypersecretion usually due to pituitary tumors, especially eosinophilic adenomas, producing gigantism and/or acromegaly. Certain cases have been reported with signs and symptoms of acromegaly, but without pituitary tumors. Serum growth hormone is elevated, and in some cases circulating GRF activity has been found. These patients may represent a hypothalamic disorder with excessive synthesis of GRF (Martin, 1973).

OTHER PORTIONS OF THE LIMBIC SYSTEM

The limbic portion of the thalamus consists of the dorsomedial nucleus and the anterior nucleus, sometimes referred to as the anterior thalamic tubercle. In addition to intercommunication with each other, with reticular thalamic nuclei, and with adjacent thalamic nuclei related to motor control or somatosensory function, each of these nuclei receives a major input from one portion of the amygdala-hippocampal system and sends output to the limbic neocortex. The anterior nucleus receives the large fiber tract from the mammillary nucleus and may receive some fibers directly from the fornix. Its output passes through the anterior limb of the internal capsule, separating the striatum into caudate and putamen, curves around the anterior horn of the lateral ventricle, and terminates along the cingulate gyrus (Yakovlev et al, 1960). The inferior thalmic peduncle carries fibers from basolateral amygdala and overlying hippocampal cortex to dorsomedial nucleus. The major projection of the limbic thalamic nucleus is to frontal orbital neocortex (Locke et al., 1961).

Portions of the midbrain usually included within the limbic system are periaqueductal gray, midbrain tegmentum, ventral tegmental area of Tsai, and the interpeduncular nucleus. The sleep related areas of locus coeruleus and raphe nuclei also have marked interactions with the limbic system via median forebrain bundle. The dorsal longitudinal fasciculus originates throughout the hypothalamus and runs through the midbrain adjacent to the periaqueductal gray and near the locus coeruleus. Many fibers communicate with these areas before descending to more caudal brain-stem regions including the salivatory nuclei, the nucleus ambiguous, and the facial nucleus. The mammillary bodies communicate with many midbrain areas, particularly with the interpeduncular nucleus. The habenula sends fibers to midbrain by means of the fasciculus retroflexus.

Major communication between limbic midbrain areas, hypothalamus and preoptic regions, and orbital and frontal neocortex is via the median forebrain bundle. Major input to this system originates from the serotonergic cells of the raphe nuclei and from noradrenergic cells of the lateral brainstem, particularly the locus coeruleus. Whereas the median forebrain bundle represents the only major ascending system of the raphe nuclei, the noradrenergic system has two outputs, one via the dorsal noradrenergic bundle to the reticular nuclei of the thalamus, especially the central median nucleus, and the other via the ventral noradrenergic bundle which joins the median forebrain system. These fibers are poorly myelinated and have only been appreciated since the development of combined neurochemical and neuroanatomical techniques (Morgane and Stern, 1973).

The limbic system also contains some elements of six-layered cortex, termed isocortex or neocortex. Limbic neocortex includes parolfactory and subcallosal gyri, the cingulate gyrus, orbital frontal cortex, and the neocortex on the medial and undersurface of the temporal lobe, including hippocampal and fusiform gyrus and possibly inferior temporal gyrus. The parolfactory and subcallosal gyri receive limbic input from the medial olfactory stria and septum, and communicate with other frontal lobe neocortical areas by means of subcortical white matter. The cingulate gyrus receives input from the anterior thalamic nucleus and communicates to other areas via the cingulum—a white matter bundle which courses along the border of the cingulate gyrus, around the splenium, to continue along the hippocampal gyrus. The orbital cortex receives input from the dorsomedial nucleus of the thalamus and communicates with the amygdala and hippocampal cortex via the subcortical white matter bundle called the uncinate fasciculus. The studies of Van Hosen and co-workers (1976) show that the cingulate gyrus receives somatosensory information from the postcentral gyrus, visual information from posterior parietal cortex, and auditory information from near Heschl's gyrus.

CLINICAL CORRELATION

The neurologist likes to correlate anatomical lesions in the brain with changes in behavior and sensation, so that he is able to translate a patient's signs and symptoms into an anatomically localizable problem which can be etiologically diagnosed and effectively treated. The neurologist most easily comprehends anatomical lesions which interfere with long tracts carrying sensations to and commands from central regions. Unfortunately, these tracts are not within the limbic system and, with one exception discussed in the next paragraph, no unilateral limbic lesion produces a chronic, permanent, nonepisodic abnormality in the neurologic examination. Certain lesions within the temporal lobe and hypothalamus produce visual field defects, not due to direct limbic damage, but rather to involvement of optic chiasm just inferior to the preoptic area, optic tract adjacent to the hypothalamus or geniculo-calcarine fibers in the deep white matter of the temporal lobe. The latter fibers—called Meyer's loop—are frequently destroyed by temporal lobectomy, producing a superior quadrantanopsia (Marino and Rasmussen, 1968). Unlike the lateralized psychological functions of the neocortical cognitive system, which assign speech to left and spatial skill to right hemispheres, functions within the limbic system are predominantly duplicated within two corresponding structures of the two sides, although we are beginning to appreciate a few exceptions which will be examined later in this book.

Unilateral lesions of the olfactory nerve, bulb, or tract produce an inability to smell substances sniffed with the ipsilateral nostril. It was long believed by neurological clinicians that odorous fumes passed from one nasal cavity to the other, possibly via the anterior cranial fossa through the cribiform plate, so that lesions of the olfactory nerve could be detected only if bilateral. The studies of Gordon and Sperry (1969) in epileptics with surgical section of corpus callosum and anterior commissure have revealed, however, that with one nostril occluded, a brief sniff of an odorous substance through the other nostril causes olfactory information to travel down the ipsilateral olfactory tract to be registered in one hemisphere only. If this is the left nostril and left hemisphere, the blindfolded subject can verbally identify the substance as discussed in the previous chapter. Gordon and Sperry (1969) found that some internal transfer could occur with prolonged intake by one nostril, but not if the open nostril was pinched shut immediately after the initial sniff.

More extensive, bilateral destruction of portions of the limbic system can produce dramatic changes in behavior, memory, emotion, and vegetative functions. Complete hypothalamic destruction causes increased eating and obesity, emotional instability with episodes of rage, lability of body temperature, and a disturbance of sleep pattern with loss or reversal of the normal circadian rhythm (Killeffer and Stern, 1970). Anterior hypothalamic destruction in man produces loss of the heat-conserving mechanisms of peripheral vasoconstriction and shivering with episodes of hypothermia when exposed to cold (Fox et al., 1970). Small lesions of the central hypothalamus can produce emaciation (Lewin et al., 1972). These patients can be mistaken for anorexia nervosa patients, but they do not show the psychiatric concomitants of this disease such as a distorted body image, the belief that emaciation represents a desirable physical condition, and a long history of preoccupation with food, cooking, and diets (Maxmen et al., 1974).

Much of our knowledge of the effects of bilateral limbic lesions comes from the neurosurgical destruction of portions of the brain in attempts to alleviate epilepsy and psychiatric disorders. Removal of one temporal lobe for treatment of epilepsy causes no emotional or personality changes. Removal of both temporal lobes causes a serious disorder of memory, which is discussed in the next section. Destruction of the anterior cingulate gyrus

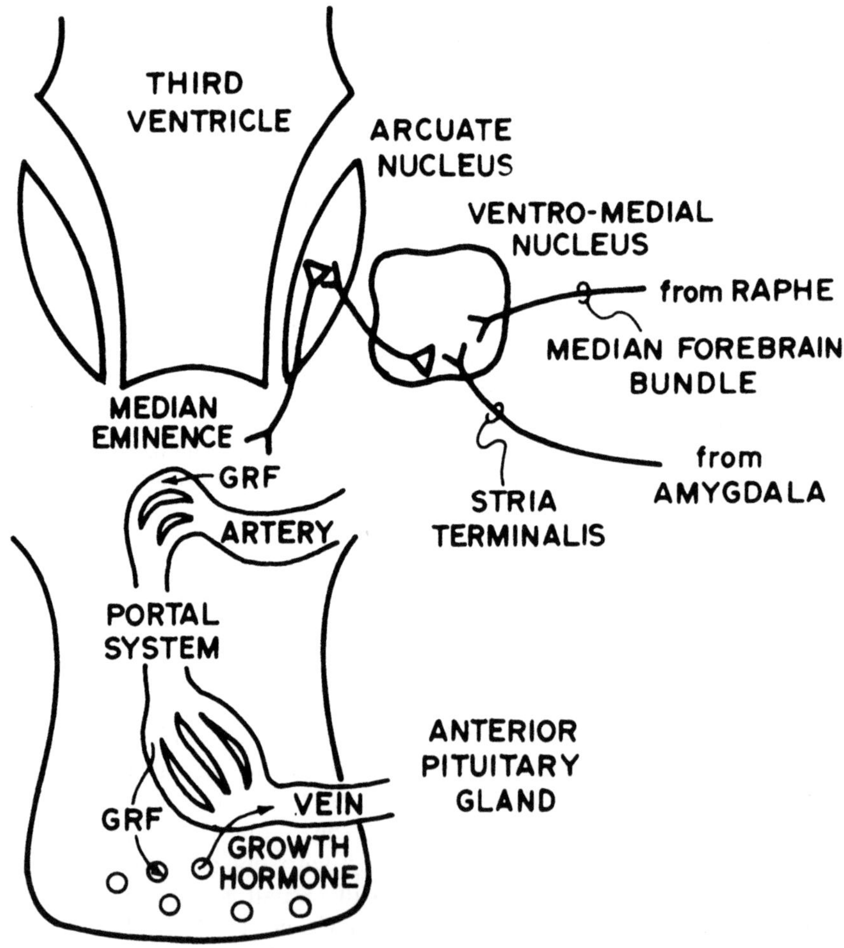

Figure 3: The limbic system influences neuroendocrine function. Control of growth hormone is a well-studied example.

decreases anxiety and obsessive-compulsive behavior (Brown and Lighthill, 1968). Bilateral destruction of amygdala decreases violent outbursts especially in epileptic individuals (Kiloh et al., 1974). Neither of these operations produces permanent memory deficits.

Limbic Memory Disorder

A very specific disorder of memory has been associated with bilateral limbic lesions (DeJong, 1973; Van Buren and Bourke, 1972). An inability to make new memories and a long retrograde amnesia characterize this syndrome. The patient appears alert, responsive, and mentally clear. He may carry on a perfectly normal conversation with the examiner on a philosophical or historical point; if the examiner is to leave and then return, however, the patient not only fails to recall the discussion, he does not even recognize the examiner. These patients are also amnestic for material which occurred prior to the onset of the limbic damage—a phenomenon termed retrograde amnesia. Those events occurring just prior to the onset of disease cannot be recalled or even recognized; remote events are well described, while intermediate events are hazily remembered. For example, a patient with bilateral hippocampal destruction might name the President as Eisenhower, yet when told Kennedy's name he might spontaneously recall the assassination. He might be able to pull the names of Johnson and Nixon out of a list but be totally unable to recognize the names of Jimmy Carter and Gerald Ford. The retrograde amnesia affects personal as well as general memories. The patient will not recognize recently acquired friends or even his wife if he has known her for only a period of months; he will, however, recognize relatives known for many years. Remote memory seems intact and the patient can frequently come up with surprising pieces of information, such as his social security number or the address and telephone number of his home where he lived many years ago. Chapter 7 reviews in detail the symptomatology and various etiologies of this startling syndrome.

A theory of memory which postulates three stages to memory formation attempts to organize our knowledge of memory pathology. While this theory accounts for all the major clinical findings, we must not be so dedicated to this or any theory that we fail to observe new findings and exceptions which can help us to devise a new theoretical construction upon which to test new as well as old facts. The postulated memory stages are usually termed immediate, short-term, and remote. However, a few workers have called them short-term, intermediate, and remote, respectively, and some psychologists use the term sensory or perceptual memory to refer to the first stage. Because of this confusion in terminology, especially in the use of the word short-term, we will use the terms surface, shallow, and deep to refer to the three stages of memory.

Actually, human lesions which disrupt memory are only clearly described for the second memory stage, the syndrome of limbic memory loss. This syndrome does not interfere with ongoing surface memory; the patient with limbic dysfunction can still follow a conversation or repeat six digits given to him at a rate of one per second. There is an inability to solidify this memory, however, an inability to place items from surface memory into more permanent stores. Retrograde amnesia is explained as an inability to withdraw items from shallow memory for transfer to the ongoing stream of consciousness. This syndrome of limbic dysfunction can be conceptualized as a disorder of transfer of information from surface to shallow storage, or vice versa. During the period of limbic dysfunction, items in surface memory are not filed, so that following neurological reconstitution, this information is forever lost and the patient is permanently amnestic for this period. It should be noted that there is some evidence that the information is actually misfiled and the reinstitution of the pathological condition that caused the limbic dysfunction will allow access to this buried material. Formally called state specific or state dependent learning, this phenomenon has been the subject of many fictional melodramas, including the first detective story in the English language, Wilkie Collins' *Moonstone*.

The first and third stages of memory are not as clearly associated with any pathological condition. No known disease process affects deep memories while leaving shallow storage undisturbed. The border between surface and shallow is fairly clear, while the border between shallow and deep is not. Some slight clinical correlation is possible with supposed disorders restricted to surface memory. Lesions in or near the primary auditory projection area of the cerebral cortex of the speech-dominant hemisphere cause a disorder of verbal abilities, which could be termed a disorder of that portion of surface memory associated with auditory verbal information. This patient is unable to repeat six digits forward. The concept of modality-specific surface-memory disorder converges with concepts of the various agnosias, amnestic aphasia, loss of memory for colors, loss of memory for faces, and other lateralized psychological functions which will be addressed in Chapters 9 and 10.

Chapter 4

Evaluation of the Patient with Organic Mental Disease

THE ART OF TAKING A HISTORY

Medical-history taking is not as simple as it superficially appears. One cannot expect the patient to know what is important and what is not. One cannot simply say, "what is your problem?" and expect all of the necessary information to be told in proper order. The information present in the patient's mind can be transferred to the physician's mind only by the art of medical interviewing. The problem is doubly difficult when the patient suffers from organic mental disease, because the organ of communication suffers from the disordered function the patient is asked about.

Many people consider Sherlock Holmes to be the greatest history taker of all time. He and Watson were always leisurely sitting around the disordered breakfast table when a breathless person desperately in trouble would come rushing in. Holmes would put him at ease and amaze Watson by telling the person a little about himself on the basis of only his outward appearance. When the person was ready to begin, Holmes would settle back in his armchair, his fingertips touching, his brow furrowed, his eyes upon the ceiling. The story comes out as though it were read from the synopsis of a novel, no extraneous information, no asides, but everything important included. However, one miniscule fact has been omitted and Holmes, silent and intent until now, asks his one brilliant question. "Did the dog bark?" "Do you have any relatives from America?" "Was Mr. Baskerville ever with the Indian Army?"

Unfortunately, Sherlock Holmes, contrary to popular belief, is a fictional character. Sir Arthur Conan Doyle, a physician, created the famous detective and based Holmes' problem-solving methods on medical diagnostic techniques. It is also unfortunate that the patient with the encapsulated and inclusive story is likewise a fiction. Patients in real life do not give the types of histories related by the people of Dr. Doyle's imagination. Some patients ramble endlessly about all of the medical misadventures of their lives. Some are so vague that they cannot even articulate their major complaint. Some patients think the doctor merely plugs in and turns on the diagnostic computer carousel; they refuse to discuss their problems beyond the barest statement. Some are so suggestible, that they agree to any symptoms the doctor mentions, from noisy flatulence to itchy teeth.

It is easy for me to recommend that you listen closely to what the patient says, and what he doesn't say. A simple platitude—listen—but how difficult it is to put into practice. Havens (1978) compares the ability to listen carefully to the patient's history to the sensitive listening to breath sounds during auscultation. The chest X-ray has atrophied our auscultatory abilities, perhaps without too great a loss to clinical medicine, much like our general technological milieu is destroying the physician's ability to hear what the patient is saying, to the great detriment of both. Burstern (1978) feels that our present medical education system actually causes deterioration of listening abilities. Speaking to medical students, he says: "Chances are you'll get so engrossed in figuring out the diagnosis that you won't listen to the patient. You'll home in on the "answer" with a series of questions like a moth flying into a light bulb, and once in a while you'll get burned. When the patient wants to tell you how he/she feels about being sick, or the possible loss of a job, or his/her fear of dying, or the feeling that he/she caused this illness, you may shut him/her up with a hearty reassurance." (As an aside one may note how the elimination of sexual reference also eliminates readability.)

THE PATIENT OF TOO MANY WORDS

The talkative, rambling patient is familiar to every physician. A specific female patient probably springs to mind but neither sex has a monopoly on this common phenomenon. This patient *must* be kept from rambling asides. As Lance (1973) testifies from his clinical experience, a patient's verbose disconnected narrative not only wastes time, it actually obscures important information and thereby dulls the physician's diagnostic cutting edge. The uncontrolled history of the loquacious patient is not unproductive, it is counterproductive.

Some patients like to detail the opinions and treatments of other physicians. "Dr. Jones gave me a little blue pill to take three times a day but . . ." Even though it may be obvious that Dr. Jones is completely out of his diagnostic depth and is merely trying to relieve symptoms, the patient respects his family physician's opinions and feels that previous treatment attempts, even though failures, produce important negative information. According to Bickerstaff (1973), English patients (the descendants of Holmes' clients) love to describe their previous medical adventures as much as do American ones: "Patients delight in describing in detail the hospitals they have been to (with dates usually accurate); the doctors they have seen (with names usually inaccurate); the detailed conversations they have had with them (with quotations usually incredible); and the treatment ordered (with results usually disastrous)."

Even though it is a natural human characteristic to want to describe and thereby relive the medical trials and tribulations one has undergone, diagnosis demands a logical separation of symptom progression from the issue of therapy. What is the natural history, and at what points have therapeutic interventions changed that history? Although some physicians abruptly cut off the patient who dwells too long on his previous therapy, I find it better to gently push the conversation back to symptom progression, although I do sometimes break right into the patient's long narrative: "Was your —— (symptom) still bothering you after you saw Dr. Jones?"

A special subgroup of loquacious historians are those who accompany a patient who has lost consciousness. As discussed later in this volume, it is absolutely essential to interview these people, yet they usually discuss their own involvement rather than the patient's. "Then I went to get a damp cloth for his forehead, then I called the ambulance, then I called his wife." Many of these individuals seem to be seeking approval for their actions from the medical authority and the most direct route back to a description of the patient's appearance and behavior requires acknowledgement of the value of these actions. A regular nodding of the head and an occasional approving grunt probably will suffice. A question that often brings out clinical description asks the observer to test his own diagnostic thinking: "What did you think was happening?" "I thought he was dead. He was blue in the face and his arms were stiff." Or perhaps: "At first I just thought he was asleep. His head was on his arm but he was breathing funny."

Severe anxiety often produces a force of speech which jumbles, rather than orders the series of events in the patient's mind. A moment at the beginning of the interview to put the patient at ease is time well invested. The ability of Sherlock Holmes to assuage his clients' anxiety may be one reason they gave such good histories.

> "Have a cigarette, Mr. McFarlane," said Holmes to the quivering and perspiring Norwood builder. "I am sure that, with your symptoms, my friend Dr. Watson here would prescribe a sedative. The weather has been so very warm these last few days. Now if you feel a little more composed, I should be glad if you would sit down in that chair, and tell us slowly and quietly who you are and what it is you want. You mentioned your name, but I assure you that,

beyond the obvious facts that you are a bachelor, a solicitor, a Freemason, and an asthmatic, I know nothing whatever about you."

THE PATIENT OF TOO FEW WORDS

A varied group of patients cannot or seemingly will not describe their symptoms. Some have a pathological respect for technology; they think the doctor need only be told the basic dysfunctioning part so he will know where to put the diagnostic machine. Some patients present limited information because of faulty memory. One can improve recall by urging the patient to

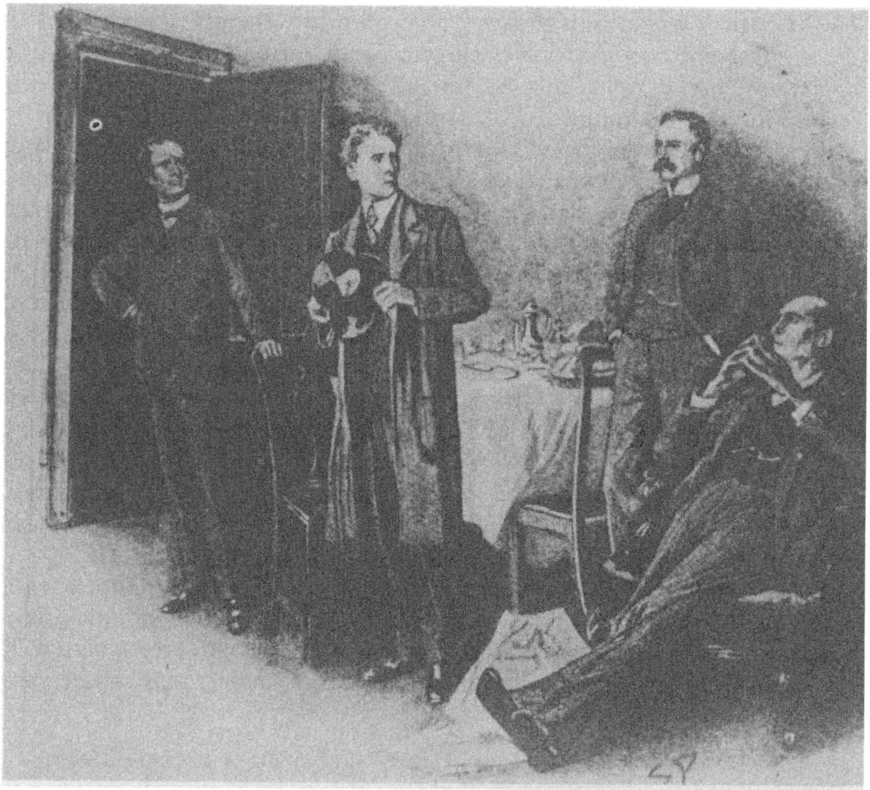

Figure 1: Mr. Holmes puts the anxious Norwood builder at his ease in order to obtain a better description of the problem. From the original drawing in *The Strand Magazine*, 1904.

go over temporally related events. "What time of day did this begin? What were you doing just before these symptoms started?" Some patients of limited intelligence have difficulty generalizing a typical attack of episodic symptoms. If the physician queries the patient about specific episodes, such as the most recent or most severe spell, a myriad of colorfully described details may emerge.

A final category of reticent patients I have recognized only in enlisted career soldiers but I imagine there is a civilian counterpart. This young man perceives the doctor as an officer; he answers the doctor's questions as directly and succinctly as possible without any real conversational exchange.

Just as anxiety produces a rambling stream in some patients, others, generally those with more severe anxiety, clam up tight (Siegman, 1978). If the reticent patient sits tensely on the edge of his chair, a few words of relaxation may improve the flow of information.

THE OVERLY AGREEABLE PATIENT

Many sick people, if not most, are very suggestible; often their desire to cooperate with the person they perceive is trying to help them overrides their critical faculties. "Are you sure so-and-so did not occur?" The doctor knows more about this than I do, the patient subconsciously feels, perhaps so-and-so did occur.

One resident used to brag he could take a history in a minute. As soon as the patient stated his chief complaint, the resident would recite for the patient two or three classical histories and ask the patient to choose the closest fitting. If the patient said he passed out, this resident would say: "There are two ways to pass out. One is like this (and he would describe a classic case of syncope) and the other is like this (and he would describe a seizure). Which one did you have?" Not many patients were independent enough to answer, "none of the above." Of course, the resident was joking, but the basic principle of humor is exaggeration of the truth, and this particular resident has been known to "uncover" historical elements from a patient which were not corroborated by a subsequent history stripped of leading questions.

Two basic methods minimize the patient's suggestibility. The first I refer to as the method of descreasing radius concentric circles. Questions precede from the more general to the more specific; the earlier in the series the symptom occurs, the more weight it is given. Suppose you wish to know if the patient's headaches are preceded by flashing lights. First you ask a completely open question: "Does anything occur before the headache?" Possible answers include the entire universe of items and events. His negative answer is followed by a fairly open question, "Do you get any warning that a headache is coming on," or, more specifically, "if you were going to get a headache this afternoon, what would be the first thing you would notice?" Continued negative answers trigger an even more specific question, "do these headaches ever affect your vision?" and next, "is there any change in your vision just before the headache?" Continued negative or nonspecific responses cause the examiner to focus his questions upon bright lights, then flashing lights, then zigzag lights. If the patient finally says, "oh, yes, I do see flashing lights before the headache," one fears this response is due more to suggestibility than to the migraine syndrome.

The other method minimizing suggestibility is only available to examiners who are capable of controlling facial expression. (The poker player who can look bored when he picks up four aces can use this method.) A series of questions contains some that will trigger important information and some that will trigger suggestibility. A question about flashing lights is followed by a question about aching teeth, and another about itchy eyebrows. Three yes answers cancel the value of the potential information about the flashing lights.

THE ORGANIC MENTAL DISEASE PATIENT

Interviewing the patient with organic mental disease is doubly challenging. One faces the same problems as with any interview, in addition, the observing and explaining organ, the brain, is the one suspected of disease.

In the majority of instances, it is necessary to interview both the organic mental disease patient and another observer, such as the spouse. Some patients experience episodic changes in thinking or behavior. Often their descriptions of their subjective feelings and observations provide great diagnostic value. Since these descriptions can be clouded by the organic mental changes which may have accompanied or preceded these episodes, it becomes essential to obtain a corroborative description by an observer. There is something ironic or paradoxical about asking someone who complains of memory loss to relate the details of his symptoms. If he could remember these details, he wouldn't be complaining. Therefore, it is essential for both the patient and another person, usually the spouse, to attempt to relate the history. One can then compare the "real" history with the patient's conception of it. For example, a patient's spouse may have noted that abnormal behavior began in mid-afternoon, while the patient remembers breakfast but not lunch, indicating temporal dissociation of amnesia and behavioral dysfunction.

The question arises whether patient and spouse should be interviewed together or separately. Being interviewed together saves time and allows observation of husband-wife interaction. As the spouse relates the onset of an episode of amnesia, the examiner can quiz the patient about elements he remembers; the exact moment of amnesia onset can thus be determined. Unfortunately, some couples cannot be interviewed together. One of the pair may answer all questions directed to the other, even mental status examination questions such as "who is the President?" One of the pair may be embarrassed to discuss behavioral abnormalities that were observed or experienced in front of the other. I recommend an attempt to interview the two together. Should the patient's spouse monopolize the conversation, or should one or both appear embarrassed, the examiner can step into the hall with the spouse while the patient undresses. This history in the hall can be amplified (or denied) by the patient when the doctor returns.

Some demented patients don't know why they are in the doctor's office or hospital. The need for the history from relatives becomes obvious. Some patients are too embarrassed to admit that they don't know why they are in a hospital, or they assume it to be related to long standing minor symptoms such as headache or backache. It is not too unusual for a medical student to stagger out of the hospital room of a demented patient with seven pages of symptoms but no inkling that the patient has organic mental disease. In rare cases, the amnesia following head injury erases the patient's memory back to a previous hospitalization for a totally unrelated condition. Using the epistemiological theory, "to name is to explain," we call this syndrome reduplicative paramnesia.

MENTAL STATUS EXAMINATION

Often, one fades from the collection of historical information to the testing of mental function. While this is operationally acceptable, even preferable, it remains essential for diagnostic purposes to separate data on how the brain is functioning at this time (the mental status examination) from the mode and rate of change (the history).

When they undress for the physical examination, many patients develop a mental set of tight-lipped stoicism. Some physicians have experienced superior results when the mental status exam is performed immediately following, or even during the history. Elements of the examination can be triggered by the patient's complaints. "You are having trouble with your memory? Let me test it a bit; repeat these numbers after me. . . ." The alert physician may note a potential abnormality of mental function by the patient's behavior and interrupt his history to pursue this. "You seem to have trouble thinking of the right words. What do you call this thing here. . . ?"

Several treatises give detailed and voluminous "bedside" tests of mental functioning (Lezak, 1976; McFie, 1976). Many physicians are so put off by the seemingly endless extent of the perfect mental status examination, that in exasperation they perform no examination at all. Strub and Black (1977) present what they call a screening mental status examination which a practiced physician can administer in 15 minutes. Even this expenditure of his valuable time may be more than the average physician can afford.

In my opinion, the mental status examination must be individualized from patient to patient based upon suspected pathophysiology. Like interviewing techniques, mental status examination is an art form. For example, a full battery of language tests would be a terrible waste of time for both patient and examiner in a patient without any hint of language dysfunction. On the other hand, testing in some detail is indicated when the patient complains of some language difficulty, has some subtle speech defect when presenting the history, or has other findings which suggest damage that might involve language-related portions of the brain.

Each subsequent chapter presents a portion of the mental status examination related to specific suspected mental disabilities. A few general remarks may be beneficial. A prerequisite for adequate mental testing is communication contact between patient and examiner. If the examiner cannot establish eye contact with a lethargic or a delirious patient, he cannot expect meaningful answers to his questions, although he can still obtain important observations from the patient's spontaneous and stimulated behavior. A second general rule is to avoid an accusatory or taskmaster tone. Just a few minutes ago, I was startled to hear a resident screaming in staccato monosyllables: "Where are you, where are you?" The frightened and obviously confused patient was frantically looking around the hospital room for something familiar for his memory to latch on to. I thought he might reply, "I fear I have fallen into the hands of the Gestapo."

THE HOSTILE PATIENT

Many patients with mental difficulties become hostile when they fear an examination will demonstrate their mental shortcomings. This hostility can be minimized by downplaying formal aspects of testing, by demonstrating a friendly and open attitude, and by approaching the problem in a way which does not threaten. Sometimes when hostility begins during the examination, it is impossible to continue at that sitting; however, if the physician is forewarned, several techniques can gather information even in the face of hostility. One technique starts out with conversation and slowly moves toward more formal testing. With the frightened patient of the previous paragraph, for example, who was not hostile but might shortly have become so, I touched him on the arm, established eye contact, and asked him his name as though it were on the tip of my tongue. Of course I didn't seek information about his name, which was written on his wristband, rather about his knowledge of his name. I then asked where he lived and what he did for a living. When I asked him how long he had been "here" he looked around without recognition and spontaneously admitted he didn't know where he was. He was now ready for deeper probing; I told him he was in a hospital because of memory troubles and before long he was describing hallucinations that the most severe questioning methods could never have uncovered.

A method I find useful with the mildly confused and obviously hostile patient I call the officialdom technique. The examiner assumes the role of some minor medical official. After correctly identifying himself, he makes an officious comment about "needing some information for our records." It is best if the patient's answers to a series of questions about name, age, wife's name, address, phone number, and social security number can be written by the examiner on an official-looking piece of paper, preferably on a clipboard. One can later compare the patient's answers to other sources, such as his social security card or the telephone book. One is justified in telling the patient innocuous lies.

Q: How long have you been here?

A: How long do you think I've been in this crummy hospital? (You've found out he knows he is in a hospital.)

Q: According to our computer summary you have been here six days. (A little lie but most patients think every hospital is somehow computerized.)

A: Your computer is really screwed up, Doc; I just came in last night.

Q: We have had a lot of complaints about the breakfast we served this morning (not true), how was yours?

The patient's answers show good memory for the past few hours. Most American patients (probably true throughout Western civilization) have had a lot of experience with officialdom, and most have concluded that the quickest way to end the ordeal is to answer the questions. When the patient finally realizes he is being tested, he may refuse to continue, but by that time the examiner has amassed a great deal of useful mental status information.

LABORATORY STUDIES

Oldendorf (1978) has presented an interesting and valuable way of looking at diagnostic laboratory studies. He imagines that each study reconstructs a map or pattern of brain pathophysiology. Each test develops an image of the brain. For example, the radionuclide brain scan measures the distribution of uptake of radioactive isotopes by intracranial tissues. In general, abnormally increased uptake represents a decrease in the barrier of passage between the lumen of blood vessels and extralumenal portions of brain tissue, the so-called blood-brain barrier (Brownell et al., 1974). Table 1 presents the various brain images constructed by several neurological diagnostic tests.

Some might include neuropsychological testing in the Table. Many clinical psychological test batteries attempt to predict anatomical localization. Usually, however, other diagnostic tests are so superior at lesion localization that psychological testing is best utilized to describe the type and quantitate the degree of psychological dysfunction, so that serial tests can record improvement or deterioration (Birkett and Boltuch, 1977).

Of course, many laboratory studies do not fit into this anatomical mode of thinking. Tests of blood components can define elements of importance to brain function through systemic effects. The lumbar puncture remains the only simple method to sample the fluid into which brain wastes are exuded.

DIAGNOSIS

Diagnostic experts commonly testify to the importance of the history in diagnosis. "The greatness of master neurologists," claims Richardson (1977), "is in large measure due to cultivated skill and meticulous care in obtaining and recording the history." Lance (1973) uses a military metaphor: "The diagnostic battle is commonly won or lost in the first skirmish." The key to diagnosis is the clinical history. Although this dictum is frequently claimed, it often finds no further use beyond pontification. In his textbook Mumenthaler (1975) uses a disability aphorism, "a blind neurologist is better than a deaf one," to illustrate this rule, but his paragraph on how to take the history is dwarfed by 31 pages on how to perform the neurological examination.

In the field of organic mental disease, failure to make a proper diagnosis most frequently results from failure to take an adequate history. The remainder of this book should prove the absolute necessity of a corroborative history from an observer when the primary history is given by someone who presently has abnormal mental function. The history alone, before the performance of any examination, permits (almost forces) the formulation of a diagnostic impression. This impression guides the performance of the mental status examination. The impression may change during that examination or during the more mechanical performance of general neurological and physical examination. The new or confirmed impression selects appropriate laboratory tests and clinical management.

TABLE 1: "Image of the Brain" as Generated by Diagnostic Laboratory Studies (adapted from Oldendorf, 1978)

Test	*Measurement*	*Reflected Pathophysiology*
Electroencephalogram	Distribution of electrical activity over scalp	Electrical activity of brain
Radionuclide scan	Distribution of isotope uptake in brain tissue	Changes in blood-brain barrier
Computed tomography	Computerized reconstruction of x-ray diffraction	Tissue radiodensity
Cisternogram	Distribution of isotope in CSF spaces	Flow through CSF
Echoencephalogram	Ultrasound reflection from intracranial structures	Position of third ventricle
Pneumoencephalogram	Distribution of air in CSF spaces	Morphology of CSF spaces
Cerebral arteriogram	Distribution of dye in blood vessels	Blood vessel position and morphology

The author has found the concept of syndrome diagnosis useful. The first stage in the diagnostic formulation is the determination of the general type of brain dysfunction without consideration of etiology. Subsequent search, sometimes with the aid of laboratory tests, attempts to define a cause which can be countered by appropriate medical or surgical therapy. Sometimes, one encounters syndromes within syndromes, analogous to the diagnostic circles within circles described mathematically by Feinsten (1967). An example might be the patient who complains of episodic confusion. Further analysis of this syndrome, based on the description of exactly what the patient does during the confusion and on the EEG findings, suggests temporal lobe epilepsy as the cause of this syndrome. But epilepsy is itself a syndrome and further etiologic analysis reveals a temporal lobe tumor. Surgery cures the benign (hopefully) tumor, the syndrome of temporal lobe epilepsy, and the more inclusive syndrome of episodic confusion. Each subsequent chapter of this book reviews a clinical syndrome; how to recognize it, how to search for its etiology, how to treat both etiology, if found, and syndrome, if no cause is found.

Chapter 5

Lethargy and Coma

LEVELS OF CONSCIOUSNESS

The term coma is difficult to define, despite the fact that clinicians seldom have difficulty recognizing it. Textbook definitions speak of lack of awareness, unconsciousness, absence of responsiveness. Sleep itself fulfills some formal definitions of coma, although its ready reversibility should separate these two conditions. Some neurologists, however, have emphasized similarities between sleep and coma and have predicted that increased understanding of the normal condition will lead to better treatment of the abnormal (Fisher, 1969; Freemon, 1978).

The journey from normality to coma is generally considered to be a downhill trip, as exemplified by the interchangeability of the adjectives deep and severe as modifers of coma description. A series of terms identify midway points on this downward slide (Table 1). The lethargic patient is difficult to rouse; he may be sleeping continuously or he may be awake but dull. In either case, however, when adequately stimulated, he can establish eye contact with the examiner and answer questions correctly, even though he may tend to drift off between questions. Obtundation is a step deeper than lethargy. The obtunded patient may mumble his name upon request but he is never fully rousable. Stupor implies appropriate response to physical stimulation without verbal interaction. Groaning and pushing away the painful stimulus is a level of consciousness above simple pain withdrawal, but both these levels are subserved by the term stupor. Most comatose patients make no response to pain, others perhaps only a grimace. Some patients in coma produce stereotyped postures in response to pain; these are often described by pseudoanatomic terms like decerebrate rigidity.

A large number of other terms are used for special subsets of patients with decreased consciousness, terms like alpha-coma or akinetic mutism, and these will be defined in this missive when they are used. Some feel that the very first stage on the road to coma can be simple sleepiness. Most call this hypersomnia, but others prefer the term parasomnia to emphasize the difference between pathological sleepiness and the student late for his lecture because he has overslept (Walton, 1977). Some use the term semi-coma to describe the patient on the borderline between stupor and coma. Attempts have been made to define an even deeper level of coma called cerebral or brain death. If the clinician can rule out poisoning; if the patient has no voluntary or reflex movement, including no spontaneous respiration; and if the EEG shows no cerebral activity, this diagnosis can be made. In some legal jurisdictions this patient is legally dead and tissues, including the normal beating heart, can be removed for transplantation (Black, 1975).

One must leave the term consciousness undefined. Great volumes have been written on this topic; for example, Jaynes (1977) devotes 20 pages to a precise definition which determines that the characters of the *Odyssey* were conscious while those of the *Iliad* were not. In the context of coma, however, everyone generally agrees on what they mean by consciousness. Paralysis is not coma because consciousness is not impaired. A man paralyzed by curare looks as if he is comatose but he is not; when he recovers he reports the events which occurred around him (and probably sues his anesthesiologist).

INITIAL EVALUATION

The student who has been taught to gather reams of information before acting has difficulty with the stepwise diagnosis and treatment so often used

TABLE 1: A Series of Terms to Describe Levels of Consciousness

Term	*Description*
Lethargic	Appears sleepy but eyes open with verbal stimulation; can answer simple questions.
Obtunded	Eyes open with physical but not verbal stimulation; can mumble "yes" and "no."
Stuporous	Groans when physically stimulated but speaks no words; pushes painful stimulus away.
Semi-comatose	Painful stimulation produces some motor response but no real attempt to remove the stimulus.
Comatose	No visible movement except seizures or abnormal posturing; no response to pain except perhaps a change in respiration or pulse.

in clinical practice and so clearly exemplified in the evaluation of the comatose patient. As soon as the physician realizes he is dealing with a patient who is in coma he rapidly, almost instantaneously, evaluates the cardiorespiratory system. The student may be interested in apneustic or ataxic breathing, but the initial evaluation answers a more basic question about respiration: Is there any? Usually when the neurologist sees the comatose patient, any life-threatening cardiorespiratory dysfunctions have been brought under control by the general physician.

The history, rather than the examination, has the best chance to give the etiology of coma. Needless to say, the history must be taken from other observors. So many comatose patients are unaccompanied that this syndrome is referred to facetiously as "found down." Sometimes valuable information can be obtained from ambulance personnel, although they usually see themselves as carriers of the wounded, not of information. Every effort must be made to contact relatives. While the history from others is taken in the same way all histories are, special attention should be paid to trauma, pre-existing illnesses including depression, and drug use. If the patient's entry to coma was not observed, then one must certainly identify when the patient was last seen and his behavior at that time.

The first step in the examination of the comatose patient is careful observation. Often when the neurologist arrives all he can see is the patient's chin and face appearing over the edge of the pressed white sheets. The sheets must be removed and the body observed, with allowance for the natural human desire to keep private parts private. If the patient is supine, one can observe an asymmetry of posture which might indicate an underlying hemiplegia. Spontaneous movements, including regular rhythmic activity which might mean seizures, and diffuse muscle twitches, often indicate a special series of coma etiologies. So-called voluntary movements may be valuable in determining level of coma.

Pupils

The size of the pupils represents a balance between sympathetic and parasympathetic input. The occurrence of one maximally dilated pupil, the other normal, means interruption of parasympathetic input usually due to pressure upon the third cranial nerve. Sympathetic interruption can occur in posterior hypothalamus, midbrain, central pons, medulla, cervical cord, peripheral sympathetic ganglia, or the ascending sympathetic chain along the carotid artery. In the context of decreased alertness, sympathetic involvement usually occurs in posterior hypothalamus, causing ipsilateral small pupil and slight ptosis. In the pons, the descending sympathetic tracts run near one another, almost in the center of the reticular formation. A comatose patient with pinpoint pupils results from a pontine tegmental lesion. The full Horner's syndrome, with severe ptosis and absence of sweating does not occur with brain lesions, but only from ganglionic or postganglionic destruction. Pupillary dilatation following painful pinching of the neck indicates a central Horner's; absence of this ciliospinal reflex indicates peripheral sympathetic block.

When a flashlight shines into one eye, both pupils contract. If one contracts and the other does not, the clinician can separate sensory defects in the visual system from motor defects in the parasympathetic system by observing the response of the opposite eye. If this consensual response is present, then light information is traveling from the retina of the "bad" eye to the midbrain and, therefore, the defect is motor. Incomplete involvement of visual input, usually in the optic nerve, produces an asymmetry of light response. Light shone in the eye on the involved side is apparently less effective in producing constriction. A teleologist might say that the pupillary-constrictor centers near the Edinger-Westphal nucleus of the midbrain interpret the light to be dimmer than the same light shone in the uninvolved visual system. By swinging the light from one eye to the other, the pupils dilate when the light is shone into the eye on the involved side and constrict when light shines into the normal side. Plum and Posner (1974) call this the swinging flashlight test; others speak of the Marcus Gunn pupil, although this finding was apparently not described by the noted London ophthalmologist of that name.

For unknown reasons, midbrain pressure produces a specific characteristic pupillary abnormality. The pupils are round and equal, large at about five mm, and completely unreactive. Many people refer to these as "fixed and dilated pupils," but considerable amounts of iris remain visible and the term dilated should be reserved for the maximally enlarged pupil seen in third nerve lesions, anticholinergic poisoning, and severe generalized hypoxia. These midposition, fixed pupils form a valuable sign, since they generally intimate dysfunction in the midbrain region. Active pupillary response in deeply comatose patients usually means metabolic coma.

Eye Movements

In most comatose or stuporous patients, the position of the eyes at rest reveals slight divergence, as though each eye were looking into the lateral visual field. This mildly divergent strabismus is the position of the eyes during nonrem sleep and would occur if all extraocular muscles were paralyzed. If the subject is arousable, then vigorous stimulation will bring the eyes together; the divergence reappears when the patient's level of consciousness again falls.

If one classifies this divergent strabismus as a "normal" or expected

finding in comatose patients, then the most commonly encountered extraocular movement defect in this type of clinical situation is conjugate deviation. Both eyes look to one side. If both eyes are tonically deviated to the left, then there is usually a destructive lesion in the right lateral pons or the left cerebral hemisphere in the frontal region. Another possibility is an irritative, usually hemorrhagic, lesion in the right cerebral hemisphere.

If the patient is not deeply comatose, the examiner should observe him closely for spontaneous eye movements. A confused or delirious patient will probably move his eyes spontaneously in all directions within a short period of time. If such spontaneous eye movements are absent, the examiner should make a special effort to have the patient follow a moving object. For patients with poor attention, a moving light may be best. Many confused patients will look at the examiner's face if he is speaking; in such cases, the examiner can use his own face as the moving object for the patient to follow.

Using these methods, the clinician can often uncover specific cranial nerve abnormalities. One of the most common is the sixth nerve palsy which is due to pressure on the brain stem, crushing the abducens nerve between the basis pontis and the clivus. In a complete sixth nerve palsy the patient's involved eye will be looking toward the nose. He may be able to move this eye laterally, but not past the midline. With incomplete abducens dysfunction, the eyes may be conjugate at rest while attempts to look to one side will see the normal eye move fully toward the nose but the abnormal eye fail to move fully laterally. A light shown on both eyes at this time will show its reflection from different points on the two pupils.

The patient who is too stuporous to allow evaluation of extraocular movement in this manner can be examined using the doll's eyes maneuver. A few years ago, the toy industry developed a doll, new for that time, that delighted young children because when the doll was turned from side to side her body and head turned but her eyes kept looking straight ahead. When these young children grew into neurologists and neurosurgeons they noted that lightly comatose patients displayed the same phenomenon. If the head is briskly moved up and down the eyes may show this same lag, though usually lesser in degree than the lag of horizontal eye movement following brisk to and fro turning of the head. One must be careful in this maneuver not to dislodge respiratory support. The doll's eye phenomenon is not present in fully conscious subjects unless they fix their vision on a specific object. While clearly seen in lethargic and obtunded patients, the doll's eyes phenomenon disappears as coma becomes deeper and midbrain reflexes are depressed.

Caloric Examination

If water at a temperature different than body temperature is put into the ear, convection currents develop in the semicircular canals. These currents

masquerade as head movement and the eyes make compensatory adjustments. The caloric reflex is transmitted from the hair cells of the semicircular canals down the vestibular portion of the eighth cranial nerve. This information about endolymph movement arrives in the lateral pons. Stimulation and lesion experiments in animals with corroborating clinicopathological studies in man have developed the lateral pontine gaze center as a valuable theoretical construct. Fibers from this region—also called the paraabducens nucleus and the PPRF (parapontine reticular formation)—connect directly to the nearby adjacent sixth nerve nucleus and, crossing the midline, travel with the medial longitudinal fasciculus to the opposite third nerve nucleus subserving medial gaze. Stimulation of the left ear by cold water causes activation of the left PPRF and, subsequently, of the left sixth and right third nerve nuclei, with slow deviation of the eyes to the left. In awake subjects, a compensatory nystagmus causes a jerk of the eyes to the right. In the comatose patient, cold water in one ear causes both eyes to swing toward the side of the stimulation without any nystagmus.

Warm water calorics are a bit dangerous, because it is possible for the water to be too hot and to burn. For cold water calorics, simply drop a few ice cubes in a small container of water and wait a minute or two. Using a syringe and short tube inject this ice water into the ear canal, first checking to be sure the tympanic membrane is intact. Some can get good results with as little as two milliliters. I use five to 10 ml keeping a towel under the ear to catch the runoff. Twenty to 30 seconds later the eyes will begin to conjugately deviate toward the stimulated side and, if the patient's level of consciousness is above stupor, nystagmoid jerks will occur in the opposite direction. If the patient appears to be deeply comatose but has caloric nystagmus, one suspects psychogenic unresponsiveness. The deviation will disappear in two to three minutes but you must wait at least five, and probably should wait 15 minutes, before testing the other side.

Absence of any reaction to cold water irrigation occurs with damage to semicircular canals, eighth nerve, or the pontine gaze center. Bilateral absence of any caloric response suggests severe brain stem involvement. A few patients develop nystagmus with cold water despite absence of vestibular function; this is thought to result from a spontaneous nystagmus stimulated by the alerting effect of the ice cold water (Becker et al., 1978).

Respiratory Pattern

Many have attempted to give localizing value to various respiratory abnormalities, but I have not been impressed that detailed evaluation of breathing is worth the amount of time invested. As mentioned, the initial question about breathing is a simple and important one: Is there any? If the

comatose patient is apneic, one must proceed rapidly to respiratory support.

Cheyne-Stokes respiration, waxing and waning of respiratory depth over a period of minutes, is common in all forms of coma and is sometimes seen in normal sleep. Most other respiratory abnormalities, such as apneutic and ataxic breathing, imply disease in the posterior fossa. In the patient undergoing rostrocaudal deterioration, these brain stem respiratory abnormalities signify worsening. Especially frequent in this regard is central neurogenic hyperventilation; the comatose patient lies for hours huffing and puffing as though he had just finished a 100-meter dash. Probably the most frequent respiratory sign of worsening coma involves gradual lengthening of the waning period of Cheyne-Stokes respiration, so that the apneic periods grow increasingly long. This abnormality is seen in metabolic disease as well as bihemispheral structural abnormalities.

Search for Asymmetries

One of the basic strategies underlying the neurological evaluation of the comatose patient is the search for asymmetries which might indicate that one hemisphere is more dysfunctional than the other. This search includes an examination of muscle tone, deep tendon reflexes, other reflexes such as the plantar response, and (should the patient's level of consciousness allow) differences in response to pain on the two sides of the body and in the blink reflex to threatening hand movements in each lateral visual field.

The patient may be awake enough to allow testing of muscle strength. If not, one can obtain some hints about a potential hemiparesis by comparing the tone of each extremity to passive movement. If an upgoing toe is present on one side, confirmatory evidence for corticospinal tract involvement can be uncovered if the abdominal or cremasteric reflexes are asymmetric—absent on the same side as the present Babinski sign.

If the patient responds to pain, the examiner has the opportunity to compare pain reaction on the two sides of the body. Even stuporous patients can sometimes reveal a hemi-hypesthesia if the examiner moves across the chest or the forehead from the hypesthetic to the normal side with a series of pinpricks. As the pin crosses the midline, the patient groans or twitches.

DIAGNOSIS

Basic Diagnostic Strategy

While various clinicians use differing methods, the most common diagnostic strategy differentiates causes of coma that are intrinsic to the brain from causes related to generalized metabolic function secondarily affecting the brain. Sometimes one refers to neurological coma versus medical coma, keeping in mind that these terms refer to etiologies and not to the best service or specialist to care for a particular patient. The search for asymmetries and other focal signs reflect the attempt to identify intrinsic brain disease.

Unfortunately, a number of patients with intrinsic brain disease do not show focal signs and, conversely, some patients with focal signs have generalized metabolic disease. The former situation results from deep seated masses, bilateral subdural hematomas, or acute blockade of CSF flow and bilateral ventricular dilatation. Most of these patients show frontal lobe signs on neurological examination. The latter situation occurs in a patient with a compensated brain lesion; the precariously compensated brain tissue is more affected by generalized metabolic disruption than normal brain tissue. This is especially common after recovery from a stroke; very minor metabolic diseases such as pneumonia produce a recurrence of the stroke symptoms which disappear with appropriate treatment of the underlying systemic disease. I recently saw a diabetic patient, receiving a bit too much insulin, who developed a hemiparesis each morning that disappeared within seconds following intravenous glucose therapy.

Despite these exceptions for which the clinician must be forever vigilant, the basic dichotomy of neurological and medical coma etiologies provides the best diagnostic strategy. In addition to the focal signs already discussed, a few other signs are of value in this differentiation. A stuporous patient who is more delirious than lethargic, perhaps with myoclonic jerks, is more likely to suffer metabolic than structural disease. A patient obtunded or stuporous, who has greater suppression of the caloric response than one would expect for his level of consciousness, probably has an overdose of depressant drugs such as amitriptyline, anticonvulsants, or hypnotics (Plum, 1978). Decerebrate posturing, defined in the next section, indicates pressure on the junction of midbrain and diencephalon, either from anatomic disease or brain swelling; in the absence of cerebral edema decerebrate posturing does not occur in metabolic coma.

The central syndrome of rostrocaudal deterioration can be mistaken for metabolic coma. This syndrome and the lateral syndrome of rostrocaudal deterioration, originally described by McNealy and Plum (1962) and codified by Plum and Posner (1974), refer to the stepwise clinical signs seen with expanding supratentorial mass lesions. A centrally placed mass causes early changes in consciousness. As the mass expands, the pupils become slightly large and unreactive; eventually all extraocular movements disappear. These pupils are called "fixed and dilated" by many, but actually they are only slightly larger than normal. These midposition, fixed pupils are very characteristic of midbrain pressure. The less common lateral syndrome produces asymmetric signs including hemiparesis, only later involving consciousness. When the mass enlargement causes uncal herniation through the tentorial notch upon the third cranial nerve, the ipsilateral pupil becomes maximally dilated and unreactive. Needless to say, the recognition of this stepwise progression leads to vigorous efforts to identify the expanding supratentorial mass and if possible remove it.

Coma with Focal Signs

If the patient demonstrates focal signs, even simple tone and reflex asymmetries, the clinician moves rapidly to an evaluation for intracranial anatomical lesions which should be attacked surgically. If the onset of neurological symptoms occurred over a period of weeks or months, a brain tumor is a possibility, although most brain tumors are diagnosed long before they produce lethargy or stupor. Chronic neurological deterioration, punctuated by the sudden onset of coma, can occur from hemorrhage into a tumor—a rather rare event except with metastatic melanoma or endotheliomatous meningioma (Goran et al., 1965). Acute onset of coma in a previously healthy person can be due to either stroke, acute brain infarction or, more likely, intracerebral hemorrhage. In the latter instance, initial therapy is mainly supportive, especially regarding blood pressure control, although occasionally surgical evacuation of hematoma can be lifesaving.

Fortunate is the clinician who has cranial computed tomographic scanning readily available; fortunate also is the comatose patient with an intracranial lesion. One must beware, however, the false attribution of omniscience to this diagnostic technique. We speak of cuts through basal ganglia or through the brain stem, but actually the pictures we are viewing are only a computed representation of X-ray diffraction densities. A confused patient was discharged from our hospital with a diagnosis of "psychological problems," mainly on the basis of a normal CT scan. He died three weeks later because of a massive, invasive glioblastoma apparently of the same X-ray density as normal brain tissue. A comatose patient showed the clinical picture of massive intracerebral hemorrhage but the radiologists claimed vehemently that the bright spots on the CT scan were metastases, since they were of the same density as calcium, not blood; autopsy disclosed the clinical impression to be the correct one. The most commonly missed diagnosis with CT scanning is bilateral subdural hematoma. This is so common that many clinicians double their search for this entity when a CT scan in an elderly person fails to show the cerebral atrophy expected at this age; a CT which is "too normal" might represent bilateral subdural hematomas at the same X-ray density as normal brain tissue. No test replaces clinical judgement.

Despite these caveats, the CT scan is the single best test for the evaluation of the comatose patient with focal abnormalities. Radionuclide scanning can be valuable, especially in the patient with bilateral subdural hematomas over one week old. The EEG is of interest in certain unusual forms of coma described in the next section, but in most stuporous or comatose patients, the EEG merely reflects the patient's level of consciousness and offers no real information regarding etiological diagnosis. Occasionally, a patient with depressed consciousness because of many seizures will show clear epileptiform activity in the EEG and anticonvulsant therapy can be undertaken. The skull X-ray is rarely of value although changes of increased intracranial pressure can sometimes be seen and a scheduled spinal tap avoided. The final fall back X-ray for evaluation of the comatose patient is still the cerebral arteriogram. While this valuable study depicts the status of the cerebral vasculature, including vessel shifts because of intracranial masses, the test cannot be performed unless the potential therapuetic benefit overbalances the risk of an untoward reaction with permanent neurological sequelae, a risk of one to two percent.

Coma without Focal Signs

Probably the most common cause of coma without focal signs is overdose with depressant drugs. Many patients attempting suicide, especially those with an hysterical personality, do not really wish to end their lives, but rather hope to create a dramatic event to symbolize the end of their previously miserable existence and their rebirth to a better world. Unfortunately, however, some miscalculate the dose. Diagnostic items of value include a past history of hysterical behavior or dramatic acts, talk of suicide, empty bottles on the person or at home, recent losses such as a death or a jilting, and knife scars on the wrist. Barbiturate poisoning sometimes produces swellings of the skin, especially on the fingers.

While depressant drugs produce the downhill slide—lethargy to obtundation, to stupor, to coma—other drugs produce delirium. Delirium with tremor, muscle twitches, and sometimes seizures is produced most frequently by the tricyclic antidepressants in depressed patients emptying their medicine cabinets, and by phencyclidine in street abusers (Burns and Lerner, 1976). Scopolamine overdose, which frequently occurs with suicide attempts or gestures which utilize over-the-counter sleeping aids, also produces delirium, as discussed in more detail in the next chapter.

Treatment of overdosage involves attempts to prevent absorption of ingested drug, to hasten elimination of the drug already absorbed, and to support vital functions until the drug is metabolized. If the comatose patient has recently ingested the causative agent, the first step is gastric lavage. If the patient is awake enough not to aspirate, lavage should be followed by ipecac-induced emesis, since this frequently extracts additional drug (Goldstein, 1969). Hemodialysis should be considered in a severely comatose patient but can usually be avoided if the patient has normal renal function. Poisoning in someone with kidney disease usually dictates some form of dialysis.

Most medical diseases when severe enough can produce coma. The majority of clinicians have developed an organized approach for the comatose patient without focal signs, not known to be a drug overdose. If the physician's practice includes experience with alcoholics, he probably administers thiamine to every comatose patient in order to be certain he does not leave a Wernicke's encephalopathy untreated. Most physicians administer glucose intravenously to each comatose patient, after first withdrawing a blood sample to measure serum glucose, just in case the coma results from hypoglycemia.

Some clinicians find a mnemonic a valuable device to aid the sometimes emotional evaluation of the comatose patient. The word *etiology* provides one such mnemonic for the etiology of coma without focal signs. The origin of this memory aid is buried in emergency room lore, but it is often attributed to the internist Hugo Weber.

OTHER COMA SYNDROMES

A series of related syndromes intrudes into any discussion of lethargy and coma. This section will consider akinetic mutism and the locked-in syndrome—two conditions which appear clinically similar but are actually totally different—as well as psychogenic unresponsiveness and the unusual picture of the EEG in so-called alpha coma. In addition, this section will include a brief discussion of the opisthotonic postures sometimes seen in comatose patients.

Akinetic Mutism

To a superficial observer (including many doctors and all medical students), this patient seems awake and alert. His eyes are open and they may even seem to follow a moving object. Except for his eyes, however, he seldom moves, although he may occasionally produce an automatic movement such as a yawn; he does not speak. The examiner is unable to get the patient to follow any spoken or demonstrated commands. The EEG shows low amplitude theta and delta waves.

The pathophysiology of akinetic mutism usually involves dysfunction of

TABLE 2: An Etiologic Mnemonic for Comatose Patients without Localizing Signs

Letter	*Key Word*	*Thought Processes Stimulated*
E	Ethanol	Consider hepatic coma, subdural hematoma, Wernicke's encephalopathy. Give thiamine.
T	Trauma	Search for scalp trauma. Was the patient found where he might have been assaulted?
I	Infection	Remember that fever and other characteristic signs of infection are absent in immunosuppressed patients.
O	Overdose	Search clothes and home for empty bottles. Was patient suicidal?
L	Longstanding illness	Look for wristband or wallet card with emergency information. If diabetic, give glucose for potential hypoglycemia and evaluate serum osmolality and ketonemia.
O	Occupational	If illness began at work, call work site to uncover exposure to chemicals or gases. Alert work force or public health authorities of potential danger.
G	Grand mal	Ask about pre-existing epilepsy or seizure-like movements.
Y	Yo-yo	Investigate previous psychiatric history. Depression can lead to suicidal overdose or can present as psychogenic unresponsiveness.

The word yo-yo is somewhat pejorative but what else begins with a Y?

medial nuclei of basal ganglia and adjacent regions of the limbic system, including the cingulate gyri and septal nuclei. This dysfunction can be produced by dilatation of both lateral ventricles secondary to obstruction of CSF flow by a third ventricular tumor (Cairns et al, 1944), by block of the aqueduct of Sylvius (Daly and Love, 1958), or, rarely, by normal pressure hydrocephalus (Hakim and Adams, 1965). Occlusion of both anterior cerebral arteries, with infarction of medial frontal and cingulate cortex, septal nuclei, and head of the caudate nucleus produces this syndrome (Freemon, 1971). Those few patients who have recovered following akinetic mutism have no memory for events that occurred when they were in this state.

A related syndrome of lethargic akinetic mutism should be mentioned. Patients with this lie with eyes closed, but can be roused with minimal stimuli such as calling their names. When roused, they show the typical clinical picture of akinetic mutism, but when stimulation ceases their eyes again close. These patients show infarction of bilateral midline and reticular thalamic nuclei (Segarra, 1970).

The pathophysiology of akinetic mutism somehow involves limbic brain regions such as medial thalamus, medial frontal and cingulate neocortex, and septal nuclei. Some have suggested the syndrome results from separation of the reticular formation and ocular centers from cognitive brain structures (Strub and Black, 1977). I think we are a long way from really understanding this syndrome.

Locked-in Syndrome

Lesions of the basis pontis interrupt motor outflow to all facial and body musculature below the eyes. This profound paralysis produces a patient who can neither speak nor move, but whose consciousness is unimpaired, as can be tested by devising a system in which eye blinks signal "yes" and "no." This condition has been called the ventral pontine syndrome, the de-efference syndrome, or the syndrome of Noirtier de Villefort, after the character in Alexander Dumas' *Count of Monte Cristo* who suffered all the symptoms of this terrifying condition. Now we usually speak of the locked-in syndrome, a term popularized by Plum and Posner (1974).

This syndrome is usually the result of an infarction in the ventral half of the pons which destroys bilaterally corticospinal and other descending motor fibers, leaving the ascending reticular activating system in the dorsal half of the pons intact. Sensory fibers are usually also spared, so that these patients feel pain but give no visible sign of this discomfort. In approximately half the cases, the lesion involves the pontine gaze center or the medial longitudinal fasciculus, so that lateral eye movements are not possible, even with caloric stimulation. Vertical eye movements and eye blinks are preserved. A similar syndrome can probably also be produced by bilateral deep hemispheral lesions damaging descending tracts although this has not been clearly described in the medical literature.

Differentiation of the locked-in syndrome from akinetic mutism predominantly involves the examiner's attempts to communicate with the patient using eye-movement code. In addition, the akinetic mute usually has associated frontal lobe signs and an abnormal EEG. Differentiation of these two conditions is not academic. The most grateful patient of my career was a man who had been considered an akinetic mute for a month before the correct diagnosis was made and I was able to establish eye blink communication between him and his family. He later partially recovered and related that hospital personnel, including physicians, had discussed his situation in his presence, assuming he was unconscious, frequently using pejorative slang terms, such as "gork" and vegetable.

Patients with both of these conditions can survive although most (in fact the great majority) die from the complications of prolonged immobility, particularly bronchopneumonia.

Alpha Coma

Most comatose patients show diffuse slowing or delta waves in the EEG. A normal EEG with well formed alpha rhythm from a supposedly comatose patient should make the clinician suspect that the patient might be locked-in or psychogenically unresponsive.

However, a rare and poorly understood syndrome of coma associated with normal EEG alpha rhythm does exist. Some call this alpha coma. Pathological examination reveals either widespread cortical lesions (usually due to generalized hypoxia following cardiac arrest) or localized infarction in the pons (Marquardsen and Harvald, 1964). In the former situation, the alpha activity usually disappears within a few days and the EEG then shows slow waves, typical of coma. The pontine lesions have an anatomical extent similar to the lesions that cause the locked-in syndrome; some cases of so-called alpha coma may actually represent simple paralysis, since the physicians did not (at least according to the published accounts) attempt to communicate with any eye-blink code (Loeb et al., 1959). In a few further cases, verbal commands were given, but the pathological specimen revealed bilateral destruction of lateral lemniscus—a lesion which produces deafness (Chatrian et al., 1964). Normal EEG, or alpha coma remains a confusing entity; only the most careful clinical, EEG, and pathological study of future cases will unravel this problem.

Psychogenic Unresponsiveness

Under this heading are subsumed severe forms of depression and catatonic schizophrenia. Differentiation from true coma usually offers little difficulty. The depressed patients look depressed and usually will begin to talk a little if the questions are slow and quiet. Catatonia is usually associated with some signs of anxiety; it is, in fact, a response to overwhelming panic. If the examiner holds the patient's arm in the air and releases it, it will hold the position for many seconds, or, in rarer cases, even for hours. The EEG is normal.

Decerebrate and Decorticate Postures

Comatose patients often assume these abnormal postures. Decorticate posturing involves mild opisthotonus, extension of the leg and foot so that the toes point to the foot of the bed, and flexed arm and wrist. Sometimes, the fingers are flexed; in other patients, they are extended. Decerebrate posturing, usually brought on by physical stimulation, involves more marked opisthotonus and extension of the arms.

The terms decerebrate and decorticate have a falsely anatomical ring. The terms derive from animal studies done during the early years of this century—surgical studies designed to produce specific anatomical destruction, but complicated by hemorrhage and irritation. Decorticate posture simply means hemispheral dysfunction. It is the posture usually seen unilaterally after a hemisphere stroke. It does not necessarily imply direct damage to the cortex; it definitely does not mean that the cortex is functionally ablated and subcortical structures are intact, in fact, just the opposite is more likely. Decerebrate posture, either spontaneous or induced by physical stimulation, usually indicates irritation, especially by acute pressure or hemorrhage at the junction of the midbrain and diencephalon.

Because these terms give false anatomical information, I tried for many years not to use them. The postures, especially decerebrate posturing, are so frequently seen, so characteristic, and so hard to describe, however, that short terms are needed. The island of Greenland is more white than green, but we can not ask all geographers to start using the "better" name Whiteland; it is too late in development of geographic and neurologic knowledge for such changes in terminology. The term decerebrate should be used as a descriptive, not an anatomic one.

Decerebrate and decorticate postures indicate anatomic, not metabolic coma. Decerebrate posturing, especially occurring episodically and spontaneously, represents a grave prognostic sign. Successful treatment is possible; a supratentorial mass lesion can be removed, or general brain swelling can be countered with steroid and osmotic agents (Brendler and Selverstone, 1970; Zervas and Hedley-White, 1972).

PATHOPHYSIOLOGY

Any discussion of the pathophysiology of coma leads immediately to the reticular activating system. The concept of the reticular activating system has proven elusive and in its original form simply incorrect. Many basic neuroscientists have discarded the concept, but it still has use for the clinician.

The anatomical extent of the brain stem reticular formation (RF) is defined by the lacy, reticular appearance of intertwined neuronal processes of the medulla, midbrain, and pontine tegmentum. Circumscribed cellular groupings such as the red nucleus and cranial nerve nuclei are excluded from RF; some diffuse neuronal aggregates with separate names, such as the nucleus reticularis pontis oralis or the raphe nuclei, are usually included within the anatomically defined RF (Broadal, 1969). RF neurons have a diffuse dendritic projection. The axon of each neuron bifurcates, descending to lower medulla and spinal cord and ascending to terminate in periaqueductal gray, subthalamus, hypothalamus, and nonspecific thalamic nuclei (Scheibel and Scheibel, 1958).

Electrical stimulation of the pontine and midbrain RF during sleep or light drug-induced coma causes fast activity to replace slow waves in neocortical EEG, and, the animal awakes (Moruzzi and Magoun, 1949). Lesions destroying midbrain RF destroy the electrographic and awakening effects of pontine stimulation and of peripheral pain stimulation; lesions which cut the classical sensory pathways, such as the spinothalamic tract, but which spare RF, do not interfere with this arousal response (Lindsley et al., 1950; French et al., 1952). These experimental findings led to the development of the concept of the ascending reticular activating system. This concept proposed the existence of a multisynaptic relation of neurons of the brain stem RF with the neurons of nonspecific thalamic nuclei which were thought to project diffusely to the neocortex. Increased excitation in the brain stem RF led, it was suggested, to increased excitation of neurons of the nonspecific thalamus, which led, in turn, to excitation of cortical neurons and wakefulness. Since sleep is known to be facilitated by a decrease in environmental stimuli—a quiet and dark room for example—sleep was thought to result from a dampening of the input to the brain stem RF, causing a decrease in activity of nonspecific thalamus and, subsequently, of cerebral neocortex (Magoun, 1954, 1963).

The concept of the ascending reticular activating system has been criticized. While withdrawal of peripheral sensory input may contribute to sleep induction, it cannot be the sole element in the development of sleep, since many active neural and neurochemical sleep-producing mechanisms have been described. Stimulation of brain-stem regions near the RF can transform ongoing cortical fast activity to slow waves; the exact opposite of the change produced by RF stimulation (Magnes et al., 1961). The nonspecific thalamic nuclei do not project diffusely to the neocortex, as postulated by the reticular activating theory in its original form; rather, these nuclei project to limbic areas, to orbitofrontal cortex, and back to the brain stem RF (Scheibel and Scheibel, 1967). They may affect the neocortex through interaction with specific thalamic nuclei. Many investigators noted quite early that environmental stimulation during nonrem sleep usually produces flattening of slow activity in the hippocampus prior to flattening in the neocortex (see the discussion following Magoun, 1954). Sometimes, a minor environmental stimulus causes fast activity to appear in hippocampus transiently, with little or no change in ongoing cortical slow activity. Environmental stimuli which awaken from nonrem sleep cause desynchronization to appear in hippocampus several seconds before fast activity replaces slow waves in neocortex. This phenomenon of hippocampal "arousal" preceding neocortical arousal occurs in many species, including the cat (Jouvet, 1967), chimpanzee (Freemon et al., 1969), and man (Freemon and Walter, 1970).

Brodal (1969) has presented the most devastating criticism of the concept of the ascending reticular activating system. A portion of his critique is directed at nomenclature. The word reticular refers to an anatomic region, while activating is a physiologic term. He objects to the juxtaposition of these words, since the full extent of the RF was not known to participate in the activating response, while arousal mechanisms certainly involved portions of the brain outside the anatomically delineated reticular structures. He also noted that portions of this system projected in a caudal direction, and, therefore, he doubted the advisability of the word ascending. He doubts that this activating system was really a neural system in the sense of the visual system or the gamma efferent system.

For basic scientists a valuable theory leads to further insights into mechanisms and function. The concept of the reticular activating system failed to predict the discovery of rem sleep and, in fact, has never been reconciled with this supposed cortical activation which occurs simultaneously with behavioral sleep. The concept failed to predict that the serotonin neurons of reticular nuclei in the midbrain raphe would project to the neocortex, bypassing the thalamus, or would have an important role in sleep onset. These failures have caused many neuroscientists to discard the concept of the reticular activating system.

On the other hand, the clinician searches for a theory that will hold disparate facts together and give his actions a rational basis. Almost all known anatomically defined lesions which cause coma involve the midbrain reticular formation. Supratentorial mass lesions seldom cause significant stupor until signs of midbrain pressure appear. The levels of consciousness observed in many patients suggest gradual suppression of reticular function analogous to a light dimming (lethargy, obtundation, stupor, coma) or brightening (with recovery, vice versa). The concept of the reticular activating system serves well for most comatose patients, but one must remember it is just that—a concept. Delirium and alpha coma are not explained. I do not think akinetic mutism is in any way illuminated by the concept of the reticular activating system, while Strub and Black (1977) suggest that the reticular formation remains connected to ocular centers, but is separated from control over cognitive portions of the brain. This seems to be little more than a tautology; the eyes are awake but the rest of the person is not.

Chapter 6

Delirium and Organic Psychosis

INTRODUCTION

Delirium is a syndrome of abnormal mental function characterized by apprehension progressing to panic, confusion to disorientation, and misinterpretation of sounds to frank hallucinations. Usually present are abnormal movements such as tremor, twitches, and jerks. Epileptic seizures can occur. Table 1 summarizes the clinical symptomatology that defines the syndrome.

Some researchers have used a broader definition of delirium, one which includes any condition characterized by clouding of consciousness—even lethargy and stupor, as described in the previous chapter (Engel and Romano, 1959). If a nurse came out of a hospital room to tell you that a patient had become delirious, you would be surprised to find that patient sleepy and hard to rouse. The term delirium implies someone who is speaking, perhaps excitedly, but whose speech lacks full coherence. For better communication among physicians as well as between a physician and a patient's relatives, it is best to restrict the diagnosis of delirium to the patient whose behavior is described by the symptomatology outlined in Table 1.

Some clinicians use the term organic psychosis as a synonym for delirium. The dictionary defines psychosis as a general term for any severe disorganization of thinking, but in actual practice organic psychosis is usually restricted to a clinical situation of abnormal excessive thoughts. Many of the same organic factors that can cause delirium acutely can, with chronic exposure, produce a delusional and disorganized patient who can be easily misdiagnosed as schizophrenic. Toxic psychosis refers to an organic psychosis due to an identifiable circulating factor, either intrinsically produced or extrinsically administered.

TABLE 1: Clinical Picture of Delirium

	Mild	*Moderate*	*Severe*
Emotion	apprehension	fear	panic
Cognition	confusion	disorientation	meaningless mumble
Thinking	racing thoughts	delusions	vivid hallucinations
Behavior	tremor	myoclonus	seizures
Autonomic	tachycardia	perspiration	fever

In practice, the use of the term psychosis frequently results in poor communication. Lay people often envision the "psychotic killer" of the cinema. I admitted to the hospital a cheerful but confused old man, unable to remember a thought for three minutes, completely harmless but with a tendency to wander. My admitting diagnosis was "Korsakov's psychosis." An hour later, I was surprised to see the man, still in street clothes, wandering around the hospital lobby. The medical nurses had refused to accept the admission because, they said, "we have no facilities to handle psychotic patients." The impasse was solved by a simple semantic expedient of readmitting the patient with the diagnosis of "Korsakov's disease."

SYNDROME DIAGNOSIS

Overwhelming anxiety, marked by apprehension, excitement, and hyperactivity, can masquerade as early delirium. Dostoevski used the term brain fever, the most common cause of organic delirium in his day, to describe many of his panic-stricken characters. By removing the patient from his relatives and sitting with him a few minutes, uncomplicated anxiety can usually be differentiated from delirium by thought content and associated autonomic and motor signs. One must avoid the natural tendency to become excited so as not to fall into the vicious circle of escalating physician and patient excitement. The more hyperactive the patient becomes, the more calm the physician should appear. The doctor should never, however, become so calm with a potentially violent patient that his guard is lowered. He should talk quietly, yawn, slump in his chair, but keep his eyes on the patient.

A common diagnostic problem concerns the hallucinatory patient. The dichotomous differential diagnosis of organic versus functional psychosis often hinges on associated findings, such as tremor and myoclonus. Sometimes, exact details of the hallucinatory thought content aid in diagnosis. While, in general, functional psychosis produces auditory hallucinations and delirium visual ones, exceptions are so frequent that predominant sensory modality is of little diagnostic import (Goodwin et al., 1971). Even some normal people may have auditory hallucinations on rare occasions, at least according to Jaynes (1977) who describes his own. The voices associated with functional psychosis usually talk directly to the patient in an accusatory or demeaning tone, while the auditory hallucinations of organic disease usually develop from environmental noises.

Severe delirium can progress to coma. Clinical value seems to accrue from attempts to visualize two pathways to the comatose state (Freemon, 1976). The more common path described in detail in the previous chapter, results from a wide variety of causes, including intrinsic anatomical lesions of the brain such as tumors or infarctions. The less common path, the subject of this chapter, is produced by a much smaller list of causes that includes drug withdrawal after chronic use, but for practical purposes excludes intrinsic brain disease. The differentiation of these two serious syndromes follows from their clinical characteristics. The lethargic or stuporous patient groans and pushes away a painful stimulus, but is grossly deficient in spontaneous thoughts and is usually devoid of spontaneous movements. The severely delirious patient lies with his eyes closed, muscles twitching, and lips moving continuously in an incomprehensible mumble. Figure 1 graphs these two theoretical roads to coma.

The only laboratory test that helps in the syndrome diagnosis of delirium or organic psychosis is the electroencephalogram (Pro and Wells, 1977). In general, the EEG is normal in the functional disorders which could be mistaken for delirium, such as mania, acute schizophrenia, or overwhelming anxiety. Since the EEG measures an aspect of neuronal function, unlike the other brain imaging techniques reviewed in Chapter 4 (see Table 1 in that chapter), one might expect EEG abnormalities in delirium. Although the EEG is often normal, especially in the more chronic organic psychoses, most acute deliria show some slowing of the background activity, often interspersed with spikes and sharp waves (Obrecht et al., 1979). Occasionally, a particular EEG abnormality can suggest, but not unequivocally diagnose, a particular disease process. One thinks of the periodic high amplitude sharp waves of herpes simplex encephalitis (Chien et al., 1977), the triphasic waves of hepatic encephalopathy, or as illustrated in Figure 2 the paroxysmal slow waves of Alfrey's encephalopathy.

A special caveat applies to the EEG of the delirious patient—a caveat both to the electroencephalographer who attempts to interpret such a record, and to the clinician who attempts to interpret the EEG report. The hyperactive and confused patient poses a great challenge to the EEG technician. Frequent and complex movement artifacts can be mistaken for abnormal electrical activity generated by brain tissue. The electroencephalographer may inadvertently report an abnormal EEG from an excited patient without

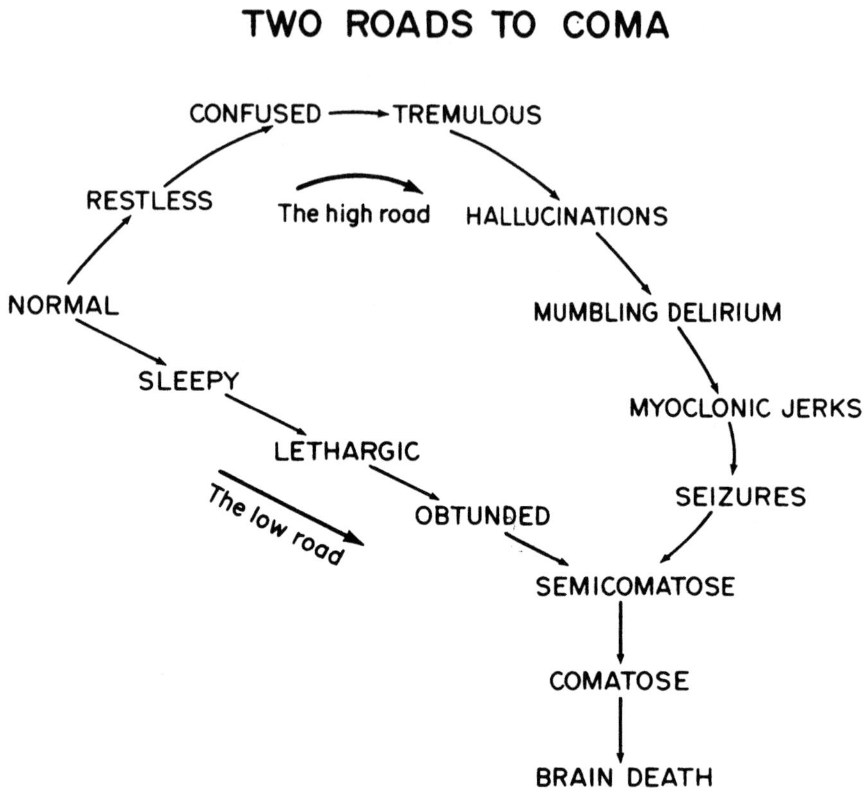

Figure 1: Clinical observations suggest that deteriorating patients become comatose by at least two different routes. The less common "high" road involves a passage through delirium.

organic brain disease or may surrender to artifact and not report intermixed or underlying true EEG abnormalities. As with all laboratory studies, the clinician must interpret the report in the context of the patient's signs and symptoms. The EEG should confirm or suggest a clinical impression, not make a diagnosis.

ETIOLOGIC DIAGNOSIS

A wide range of conditions can produce delirium. These causes generally fall into the four main categories of infection, metabolic abnormalities, intoxication with a limited number of drugs, and withdrawal of a larger number of drugs after chronic use.

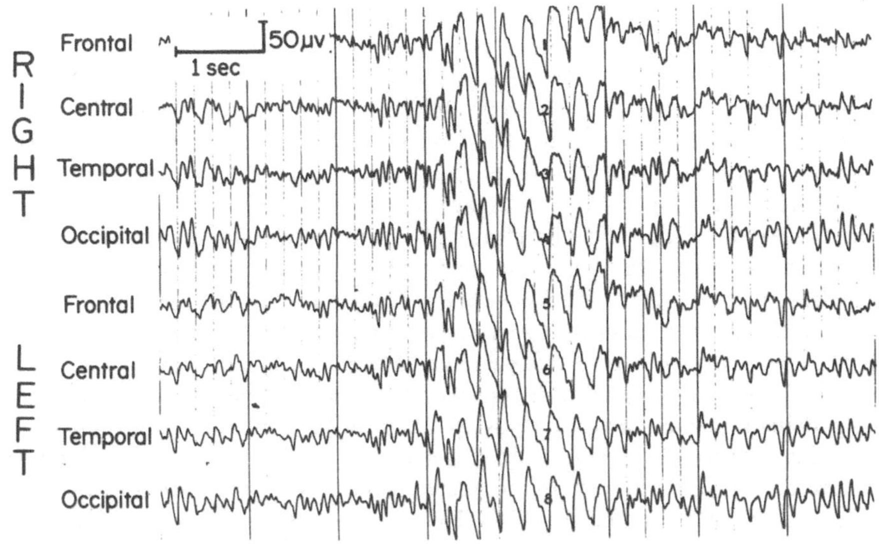

Figure 2: A burst of slow waves intermixed with sharp waves in this confused hemodialysis patient suggests the diagnosis of Alfrey's encephalopathy, sometimes called dialysis dementia.

In the pre-antibiotic era, infection was the most common cause of delirium. Direct infection and inflammation of cortical brain tissue—the syndrome of meningoencephalitis—frequently produces delirium. Common causes of delirial brain inflammation include tuberculous meningoencephalitis (Williams and Smith, 1954), subacute sclerosing panencephalitis (Ohya et al., 1974), infectious mononucleosis (Raymond and Williams, 1948), herpes simplex encephalitis, mumps encephalitis (Keddie, 1965), and etiologically undefined viral encephalopathy (Wilson, 1976). Malaria is particularly prone to present with delirium (Wintrob, 1973) or subtle mental changes (Koranyi, 1976). A small percentage of individuals with falciparum malaria can develop a prolonged organic psychosis (Blocker et al., 1968). A delirious mental state can also occur with systemic infections, especially gram negative bacterial infections with endotoxinemia. A recent epidemic of typhoid fever produced delirium in two-thirds of the cases (Osuntokun, 1972).

Common metabolic disruptions can produce the delirium syndrome. These include hypoglycemia, hypocalcemia, chronic liver failure, and chronic renal failure. A few patients on chronic hemodialysis treatment for renal failure develop an encephalopathic clinical condition, which usually progresses to delirium within a few weeks. This condition, called Alfrey's syndrome or dialysis dementia, is thought by many to be related to aluminum accumulation in the brain (Dewberry et al., 1979). An hallucinatory condition can occur with a certain degree of generalized hypoxemia; World War II pilots with primitive oxygen equipment sometimes had mental changes at high altitudes. Hypoxic delirium is, however, rarely seen clinically. Other medical conditions frequently associated with acute hallucinosis include porphyria, pancreatitis (Schuster and Iber, 1965), and decreased osmolarity and hyponatremia associated with inappropriate secretion of antidiuretic hormone (Fowler et al, 1977). More chronic metabolic disruptions which can result in toxic or organic psychosis include Addison's disease (Cohen and Marks, 1961), Cushing's disease or syndrome, thyrotoxicosis, the cerebral form of systemic lupus erythematosus (Brandt et al., 1975), and Wilson's disease (Scheinberg and Sternlieb, 1975).

Overdosage with certain drugs, both therapeutic and "social," can produce delirium. Many drugs purposely taken for their mental effects can, even in slight overdosage, result in the full delirium syndrome. The most famous of these is LSD, but others include cocaine, mescaline, and intravenous amphetamines (Logan et al., 1975). Even marihuana can produce hallucinations and panic in the unwary, particularly in the elderly (as, for example, in experimental therapy for glaucoma). Phencyclidine overdosage produces an organic psychosis resembling acute schizophrenia (Allen and Young, 1978).

Several therapeutic agents can also produce delirium. Overdosage with atropine or scopolamine was at one time very common and still occurs following suicidal attempts with nonprescription sleeping pills (Bernstein and Leff, 1967). The old description of this clinical syndrome, while very catchy, is only partially accurate: "hot as a hare, red as a beet, dry as a bone, blind as a bat, and mad as a wet hen" (Hollender et al., 1978). Intravenous physostigmine regularly (although sometimes only temporarily) reverses the delirium caused by scopolamine or other anticholinergic agents (Heiser and Gillin, 1971), including the centrally acting anticholinergics used in the treatment of parkinsonism (Black and Woollacott, 1974). The delirium of tricyclic antidepressant overdosage must partially involve cholinergic blockade, since it also can be countered by physostigmine (Burks et al., 1974). Delirium frequently complicates overdosage with levodopa, suggesting that excess dopamine may also participate in the neurochemical pathogenesis of this syndrome. Parkinsonism patients with dementia are much more likely to develop delirium following levodopa treatment than those without dementia (Celesia and Barr, 1970). The dopamine agonist agents being developed for the treatment of Parkinson's disease can also produce delirium and toxic psychosis (Serby et al., 1978). Very high overdosage with amantidine, which may act through a dopaminergic mechanism, can also cause the delirium syndrome (Fahn et al., 1971). Other drugs that frequently produce delirium or toxic psychosis include digitalis (Lely and van Entner, 1970), lithium, cimetidine (Schentag et al., 1979), high dosage intravenous penicillin, and certain other antibiotics (Byrd, 1977).

Destruction of brain tissue by infarction is a rare cause of delirium. In such cases, the infarction always involves limbic cortex (Medina et al., 1974). Brain tumors never cause delirium, but can rarely, if they impinge upon limbic system, produce a chronic organic psychosis (Malamud, 1967). Many case reports of brain diseases simulating schizophrenia clearly represent other syndromes, such as dementia or aphasia (Thompson, 1970). The so-called epileptic psychosis is a special problem reviewed in Chapter 11.

The most common identifiable cause of delirium is drug withdrawal. A wide range of drugs can produce this syndrome when abruptly discontinued after chronic use. These include the barbiturates, the benzodiazepines (Debard, 1979), and most other drugs with CNS depressant properties. The delirium which follows alcohol withdrawal is so common it rates a special name and a separate section of this chapter.

DELIRIUM TREMENS

The DTs represent a common example of the delirium syndrome. The characteristic natural history can be ameliorated by pharmacological therapy.

The first clinical descriptions are found in the works attributed to Hippocrates.

> Laerian was seized with fever after drinking. On the third day (after cessation of drinking?): acute fever, trembling of the head particularly of the lower lip, after a while convulsions, complete delirium, an uncomfortable night.

The first to use the term delirium tremens and to relate the syndrome to alcohol withdrawal was Thomas Sutton. His 1813 pamphlet (reprinted in 1941) differentiated the DTs from infectious delirium and suggested their high incidence in his Sussex practice followed from the low cost of smuggled taxless liquor.

Although a few experts feel that direct alcohol intoxication or liver disease may contribute to the development of DTs (Kramp and Rafaelsen, 1978), the major pathogenic factor is undoubtedly the abrupt withdrawal of alcohol following chronic use. Isbell and his colleagues (1955) actually produced DTs in normal volunteers who maintained daily alcohol intake for several weeks. The clinical studies of Victor and Adams (1953) showed that a series of symptoms had a regular temporal relationship to cessation of drinking. The first few hours are characterized by tremor, but no abnormal mental changes. After about 24 hours of abstinence, the seizure threshold falls to its nadir; the subject may experience a single generalized tonic-clonic convulsion. In a minority of individuals, several seizures occur within a period of a few hours. With or without anticonvulsant therapy, these do not recur as the withdrawal syndrome progresses. The patient appears normal on the second and third day, then enters the danger period for the development of the delirium tremens syndrome. During this day between alcohol withdrawal seizure and DTs, the physician must decide if the alcoholic is serious about rehabilitation. If he is, the physician can immediately begin pharmacological therapy to lessen the intensity of the delirium to come; if not, immediate hospital discharge back to the alcoholic environment may prevent further progression of the withdrawal stages, hopefully aborting the life threatening occurrence of the DTs.

Another alcohol withdrawal syndrome occurs on the first day of abstinence. Called acute alcoholic hallucinosis, this entity involves very clear auditory hallucinations in the absence of other symptoms (Victor and Hope, 1958). Many experts claim this entity is rare, but while few alcoholics complain of this phenomenon as it occurs, many will describe it in retrospect. For many patients, the voices are not particularly bothersome; they do not threaten, insult, or give orders. In other cases, however, the voices offer derogatory remarks about the patient, sometimes one particular insult voiced repeatedly. It is important not to confuse the isolated auditory hallucinations of acute alcoholic hallucinosis with the more vivid and frightening hallucinations associated with tremor and perspiration that make up the syndrome of delirium tremens.

Which alcoholics are most likely to experience these withdrawal syndromes? The most severe binge drinkers undergo some or all of these withdrawal symptoms on repeated occasions. Clinical observation suggests a personal idiosyncratic aspect repeated in each subsequent withdrawal period, complicated by a general worsening. Animal experimentation corroborates the view that each withdrawal experience is more severe and more easily induced than the previous one (Baker and Cannon, 1979).

Especially terrifying is the first episode of DTs. The heavy drinker not known to be an alcoholic may develop DTs when removed from his usual environment; the physician must be especially alert to this problem in the hospitalized patient. An EEG technician, known to be a heavy drinker, but who rarely missed a day of work, was admitted to the hospital with a broken arm. When I visited him, he was sweating profusely and talking excitedly to invisible people. This phenomenon had not been noticed by his orthopedic surgeon.

EVALUATION AND TREATMENT

In the initial evaluation of the excited and apprehensive patient with apparently crazy thoughts, one should consider, if just for a moment, that the paranoid delusions might be based on fact. Remember the case, probably aprocryphal, of the man who thought his relatives were planting dynamite in his basement. Two weeks of intensive in-patient psychotherapy overcame this delusion, but his homecoming was marred by a fatal explosion.

For the patient who presents with delirium, the history taken from friends and relatives attends particularly to his drug and alcohol use. Of course, the patient usually minimizes recent use of alcohol or social drugs, but sometimes spouse or friends also deny such use. Apparently, they fear the doctor will reject the patient as a loser who brought his symptoms on himself.

When the patient cannot or will not participate in some portion of the physical examination (usually some insignificant portion like vibratory sensation), some physicians give up. They label the patient "uncooperative" and blame the subsequent inadequate evaluation on the very delirium they are trying to evaluate. Most of the important differential diagnostic findings can be observed without any patient interaction at all—such items as perspiration, hyperactivity, tremor, myoclonic jerks. Those few portions of the exam which require the patient to sit still for a moment can usually be obtained by cajoling, confrontation, or occasionally trickery.

Etiologic considerations usually require clinical laboratory evaluation. Most metabolic causes of delirium are easily delineated by associated findings or standard laboratory measurements. If a specific infectious or metabolic etiology for the delirium is uncovered, specific therapy begins immediately. Antidotes are available for a few drug-induced deliria, but, in general, most drug-induced, drug-withdrawal, or idiopathic deliria are treated by general measures until natural restoration occurs.

The first principle of treatment of the delirious person is to protect the patient from himself. The use of restraints is always distasteful (Guirguis, 1978), but the patient who appears to be only mildly disoriented may unexpectedly attempt to escape from a hallucinated horror. In the past few years, our hospital has seen two patients with DTs crash through locked windows. Paradoxically, the one who jumped from the fourth floor hit an awning and survived, although he lost his spleen; while the young man who jumped from the second floor struck concrete steps leading to the basement and was killed. Mildly delirious patients may actually request restraints because of their own expectations of worsening hallucinations.

The second principle involves pharmacotherapy of the delirium syndrome. Unfortunately, most deliria do not respond to a specific antidote and the physician must counter hyperactivity with a depressant drug. Since delirium tremens is the most common delirious state, several controlled studies have compared potential therapuetic agents (Table 2). None appears better than chlordiazepoxide, given at a rather high dose until the patient is calm. Should he become sleepy or lethargic the dose is decreased.

TABLE 2: Controlled Studies on the Chemotherapy of Delirium Tremens

Drugs Compared	*Initial Dose*	*First Day Maximum*	*Number of Patients*	*Study Design*	*Superior Agent*	*Study*
Diazepam Promazine Chlordiazepoxide	30 to 60 mg po 75 to 150 mg po 75 to 150 mg po	180 450 mg 450 mg	103	Rotation allocation	Chlordiazepoxide	Chambers and Schultz (1965)
Chlordiazepoxide Chlorpromazine Hydroxyzine Thiamine (only)	50 mg IM 100 mg IM 100 mg IM 100 mg IM	200 mg IM 400 mg po 400 mg IM 400 mg IM	537	Random allocation, double blind (VA cooperative)	Chlordiazepoxide	Kaim et al. (1969)
Paraldehyde Diazepam	10 ml rectally 10 mg IV	Repeat until calm	34	Random allocation	Diazepam	Thompson et al. (1975)
Diazepam Barbital	20 mg po or IM 500 mg po or IM	200 mg 5000 mg	91	Random allocation, double blind	Barbital	Kramp and Rafaelson (1978)

The third principle is to treat complications as they arise. In delirium tremens, the physician will probably administer thiamine and other vitamins, not because the DTs are due to vitamin deficiency, but because these alcoholic patients often have associated nutritional deprivation. It is especially important to watch for fever. Although this can result simply from autonomic hyperactivity, it is usually due to underlying disease that is amenable to therapy. Rose and co-workers (1970) found 27 of 33 DT patients to be febrile. Careful evaluation showed that 14 of these patients had pneumonia, two had pancreatitis, and seven had fever secondary to severe dehydration. The physician must also check for complicating electrolyte imbalance, especially hypokalemia (Vetter et al., 1967).

More chronic organic psychoses need a similar detailed laboratory evaluation of liver, kidney, and endocrine function. Organic psychosis responds to dopamine antagonists, like the phenothiazines, as well as does functional psychosis. Most psychiatrists prefer haloperidol because many of the same basic disease processes which produce organic psychosis lower seizure threshold and phenothiazines might induce a clinical seizure.

Despite full evaluation, many delirious patients never have a specific cause uncovered. In other patients, delirium is associated with several factors, no one of which alone adequately explains the mental symptoms (Lipowski, 1967). An especially common association is delirium and dementia. The degree of metabolic dysfunction which would not affect the normal brain can send a mildly demented person into a florid delirium. Perhaps the demented individual has less neuronal reserve to handle either a psychologic or metabolic disruption. After an unexplained delirium clears, the alert clinician considers the possibility of an underlying dementia.

PATHOPHYSIOLOGY

Attempts have been made to explain the symptomatology of delirium. On the behavioral level of description, delirium has been called a "psychoma" analogous to tumorous overgrowths, like carcinoma or sarcoma. The suffix "oma" is meant to emphasize uncontrolled excessive production of thoughts, analogous to malignant growth of tumor cells. Psychoma is an interesting term, but it actually explains nothing.

Since delirium is rarely due to an anatomical lesion which destroys brain tissue, attempts have been made to explain delirium in neurochemical terms. Scopolamine often produces a delirium which is readily reversed by physostigmine. Cholinergic blockade can produce the limbic memory disorder described in Chapter 7, and some have suggested that scopolamine delirium is the panic which sets in when one becomes aware of the inability to make new memories associated with frightening physical symptoms such as tachycardia. Cholinergic synapses are plentiful throughout the brain and these two symptom complexes—delirium and memory loss—may be due to effects of different dosages on different circuits. For example, a low dose of physostigmine can awaken a person from drug-induced coma, while a higher dose will make a person lethargic and even induce coma, presumably by affecting different synaptic connections in the midbrain reticular formation (Avant et al., 1979). Delirium caused by excessive brain dopamine has already been discussed. Dopaminergic terminals are plentiful in limbic neocortex (Hokfelt et al., 1974); perhaps an imbalance of acetylcholine and dopamine in limbic system underlies delirium by mechanisms similar to their imbalance in basal ganglia, which produces movement disorders (Spehlmann and Stahl, 1976).

Of all the chemical agents which can produce delirium, the cardiac glycosides have been studied in greatest detail. These agents have actually been used as tools to study the action of the membrane enzyme which breaks down ATP in order to obtain energy to pump sodium out of the cell and potassium into it. Inhibition of this enzyme will lower the resting membrane potential, lowering the threshold to neuronal firing. In neurophysiological terms, this is called increasing neuronal excitability. A more excitable neuron, strategically located within the brain, might produce a more excitable person.

Another attempt to explain the pathophysiology of delirium supposes that the brain has an intrinsic mechanism functioning to overcome the effects of a depressant drug; the withdrawal of this drug after chronic use produces an overaction of this now unbalanced mechanism. Figure 3 is a graphic representation of this theory. Somewhere in the brain, location or locations unspecified, some type of neuronal action produces a neuronal response which, in turn, produces a specific behavior. A depressant drug blocks or dampens this response. Through a negative feedback mechanism, the neuronal system notes the decreased effect and makes internal changes to counteract the neuronal suppression. If the suppressing agent is abruptly withdrawn, the now unopposed increase in activity at the input portion of this neuronal mechanism produces excessive activity at the output portion, thereby causing a behavioral change which is the opposite of the initial effect of the drug. The most clearly described behavioral example of this hypothesis concerns the rem rebound which follows withdrawal of a drug which suppresses rem sleep (Freemon, 1975). Perhaps the excessive autonomic activity and the wild uncontrollable thoughts which characterize delirium can result from a similar mechanism. Treatment could theoretically involve attempts to hasten the feedback process whereby the pathological output from this neuronal system is recognized and the input which had been amplified to overcome the depressant barrier is returned to its normal level. Unfortunately, this hypothetical system has no known anatomical or neuro-

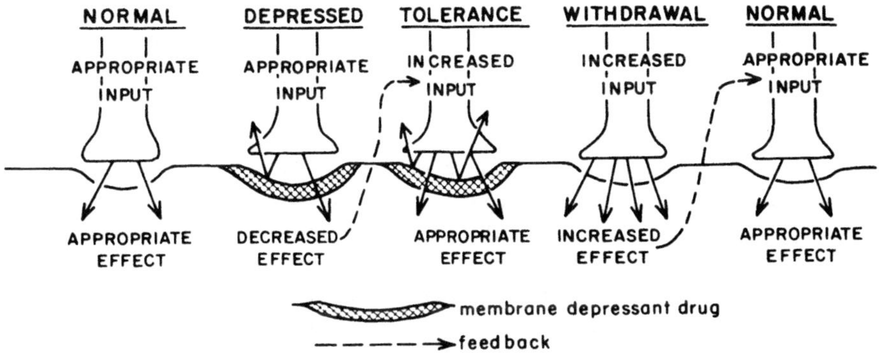

Figure 3: Perhaps the tremors, myoclonus, seizures, and delirium of a drug withdrawal state result from the unopposed hyperactivity of a neural system which had become adapted to a depressant barrier.

chemical basis, therefore, pharmacological therapy simply involves a reinstitution of the depressant barrier and a slower withdrawal.

ILLUSTRATIVE CASES

A few personal cases flesh out these bare bone facts. A hospitalized truck driver with heart disease was walking around the halls naked the night after being admitted. When asked the next morning if anything unusual had happened he replied, "I expect a little noise in a hospital, Doc, but you went too far when you rolled that grand piano into my room." He had just been started on digitalis and his EKG showed evidence of digitalis toxicity. He probably had "digitalis delirium." He later admitted to using amphetamines to keep awake during cross-country hauls, so an element of amphetamine withdrawal may have contributed to his mental aberration. Adjustment of the digitalis dosage was followed by normalization of his mental status.

The most vivid hallucination I ever encountered was described by a woman with acute intermittent porphyria. She related that she was sitting in her hospital bed, listening to the telecast of a hockey game on another patient's television set (she could not see the screen). She had been surprised when the announcer reported the arrival of the President of the United States as a spectator. Later, a fight broke out among the opposing hockey players, spilling over into the spectators' boxes. Before anyone could stop it, the President was struck and killed by a hockey stick. She had sat upright, terrified by what she was hearing and amazed that the other patients and visitors in the room did not seem excited. She knew she suffered hallucinations, so said nothing until I saw her the next day. The newspaper indeed reported that a hockey game had been televised, but the President was not a spectator. With relief, the patient accepted the unreality of her experience; yet a portion of her mind could not erase the thought that another President had been assassinated in office.

When an intern, I reported two patients with delirium developing during the course of hospitalization (Freemon and Drake, 1967). A patient with renal disease became water intoxicated. His continuous long scream was interrupted only when he paused to take a breath. He stopped screaming long enough to walk to the eleventh floor window and say, "If I jump out this window I will live forever!" Needless to say, he was restrained. When the hyponatremia abated, he recalled his abnormal thoughts; he even chuckled when he said, "I had the strangest idea last night; I felt that if I jumped out the window I would live forever." The second individual was mildly demented because of many head injuries. He became confused at night, extremely boisterous and belligerent. During the day, he actually requested that he be restrained at night so that his "crazy" thoughts would not cause him to hurt himself or others.

Just a few days ago a medical student asked me to see a patient whom he thought was not thinking clearly. The man was sitting in his hospital bed, sweaty, tremulous, wide-eyed, and apprehensive. I was speaking to him very calmly about things in general, when he suddenly turned toward the blank wall and shouted very loudly, "Will you guys cut out that racket!" When asked what they were doing, he replied something about hooking up a caboose in a railroad yard. Any further description of his hallucination was squelched when the student broke out laughing. The man was a heavy drinker and it was thought that his actions probably represented DTs. The delirium lasted over a month, gradually changing to dementia, so that the diagnosis of DTs was not tenable. This delirium, like so many, was never explained.

Chapter 7

Amnesia

INTRODUCTION

Memory loss for specific items, an accentuation of the normal forgetfulness which afflicts us all, may be the initial symptom of a wide variety of medical, neurological, and psychiatric syndromes. True amnesia is a global forgetting of all events occurring over an identifiable time span. This restricted syndrome, defined by its clinical characteristics, is caused by reversible dysfunction of certain portions of the limbic system. The pathophysiology of this disorder has been considered in Chapter 3.

When evaluated after recovery, the patient with amnesia has a blank period of definable onset and offset. Usually, he has no recollection at all for the events which occurred during this missing period. If the clinician examines the patient during the amnestic spell—the time for which he will later be totally blank—he will find him unable to make new memories. He can remember items for a few seconds; he can, for example, repeat a six-digit number. But if his attention is diverted, the material in his ongoing stream of consciousness disappears forever. In addition, this patient cannot recall events of the preceding few years. Excellent reviews of the semiology of amnesia have been offered by Symonds (1966) and Benson (1978).

Does this global form of amnesia have a special name to separate it from loss of memory for words, faces, or other specific facts or items? Some call it the amnestic-confabulatory syndrome, although only a minority of patients actually confabulate. Some call the syndrome transient global amnesia, but most restrict that term to a more specific entity. Some call it Korsakov's disease, especially when the limbic destruction and memory deficit is permanent, but most clinicians restrict this term to a specific etiology—thiamine deficiency. A few neuropsychologists call it the disorder of the second stage of memory, but this is too long to be a name and also commits us to a theory. I like the term limbic memory disorder since the histopathology involves limbic structures.

The most common cause of this amnestic syndrome is blunt head trauma. This post-traumatic dysfunction of memory gives us such terms as anterograde and retrograde amnesia. A consideration of this common condition gives us a basis for comparison with other forms of transient limbic memory disorder.

POST TRAUMATIC AMNESIA

The syndrome of post-traumatic amnesia follows a blow to the head of sufficient force to produce coma, but not so forceful as to penetrate the skull. This patient just awakened from coma appears normal and alert to a superficial observer. This alert appearance of recovery is deceiving, however, because the patient is actually experiencing a characteristic severe ongoing memory dysfunction. He not only fails to recall the accident, but has a memory deficit for months, even years, preceding the accident. In addition, he cannot make new memories. He reacts appropriately when the doctor tells him about the accident, but a few minutes later he has forgotten this conversation and, in fact, has also completely forgotten the doctor. Reviews of post-traumatic amnesia have been offered by Russell and Smith (1961) and by Schachter and Crovitz (1977).

The memory loss for events before the trauma, so-called retrograde amnesia, can be illustrated with an anecdote. A medical student was thrown from a motorcycle. When he "awoke" in the hospital room his parents were with him. As they were explaining to him what had happened, the door flew open and his flustered young bride of a few weeks rushed into the room. She leaped into his hospital bed and caressed him, expressing her relief that he had not been injured. After several minutes of love and reassurance, the wife left and the medical student turned to his mother and asked: "Who is she?" His retrograde loss had taken him back before he married or even met his wife, so he did not recognize her.

The second deficit, the inability to make new memories, can also be illustrated with a true story. Whereas the previous anecdote was related to me by the medical student after he had fully recovered, I personally observed the events of this anecdote. A patient with ongoing amnesia got the idea that he needed to leave the hospital. I actually saw the intern explaining in detail to the patient why continued hospitalization was necessary. With precise logic, the intern got the patient to agree to point after point until the patient reached the inescapable conclusion that he had to stay. The intern was beaming with the satisfaction of a good doctor-patient relationship as the patient went back to his room. However, the intern was shattered when the patient was back at the nurses' station a few minutes later, again demanding hospital discharge. The patient, of course, did not recall the brilliant logic and even treated the intern as a stranger when the whole explanation began again.

In the vast majority of instances, this post-traumatic amnesia will disappear. The alert patient who is apparently normal will convert to an individual who actually *is* normal. The mechanism of this conversion is totally obscure; some people speak of reconstitution of temporal lobe limbic pathways disrupted by a shearing force. Even the phenomenology of this recovery is unclear. One sign of improving memory is a shrinking of the period covered by the retrograde amnesia. In some cases, the patient seems to make several transitions between normal memory function and the amnestic state so that in retrospect he recalls patches or islands within his period of amnesia.

The memory of the recovered person is entirely normal. He may have elements of the post-traumatic syndrome, such as headache and easy irritability, but his memory is faultless except for a complete and total amnesia for the period of the ongoing or anterograde amnesia. The medical student described previously did not recall the episode when he did not recognize his wife, he only retold his parents' story. Frequently, but not always, this period of permanent amnesia includes only a few seconds or minutes preceding the trauma. This shrunken or truncated retrograde amnesia explains how a victim can claim he never saw the opposing vehicle in a head-on collision. When discussing details of an accident, the clinician should attempt to separate what the patient relates from his own personal knowledge from what he has pieced together from other sources.

Attempts to improve memory function during the period of ongoing memory deficit are futile. Hypnosis and amobarbital interview techniques, so effective with psychogenic amnesia, have only the slightest effect on post-traumatic amnesia (Russell and Nathan, 1946). Occasionally, a case report claims improvement following administration of a pharmacological agent, but lack of controls and the natural tendency of the disorder to improve confound interpretation (Hooshmand et al., 1974). Temporary improvement in memory may follow intravenous injection of the cholinergic agent physostigmine (Drachman, 1977).

The amnestic syndrome can follow head trauma which does not produce unconsciousness. This is especially common in American football players, among whom it is called "the ding." Evaluation of these players shows a brief retrograde amnesia and the inability to make new memories (Yarnell and Lynch, 1970, 1973). The television football addict can actually see this syndrome occur about once per game. An offensive player runs the wrong play because he cannot recall the play called in the huddle. He is called to the sideline and briefly examined by the assistant coach. If the bewildered player looks toward the opponents' end of the field, one can imagine that the coach has asked the name of the opposing team. The viewer now recalls the severe trauma experienced by the player on the previous play.

SYNDROME DIAGNOSIS

The symptoms are completely different, depending upon whether one examines the patient during or after the period of transient limbic dysfunction. During the period of ongoing memory loss, the patient's retrograde amnesia causes him to live at some time (usually some vague time) in the past. His age is too young, his children are too young, the President is someone from the past. Each clinician will develop a few questions for his own patient population. When I practiced in Milwaukee I used a question about "your favorite ball player active today." Eddie Matthews, who had retired many years before, was a response of many of these patients. Here in Nashville a similar question is not possible because of a lack of notable sports teams. Since this is Music City I might develop a question about country western music stars but my own lack of historical knowledge inhibits interpretation. One can also ask about current news events. For example, as I write this a question about Three Mile Island elicits from a normal patient a facial expression of recognition and a discussion of Pennsylvania's search for a new capital. You, reading this years later, may or may not recall the nuclear accident; the patient with a retrograde memory loss certainly will not. One can test ongoing memory by placing three items in one's pocket. If the patient shows signs of inattention, the clinician must be doubly sure that the patient recalls these items after a few seconds. After the passage of several minutes, the amnestic patient will not only have forgotten the items, he will have forgotten the entire concept.

Examined after reversion to normal, the patient will have a blank period lasting from hours to weeks. The clinician should try to define the time of onset and offset of the anterograde memory loss. Where was he when he "woke up?" What is the last thing he remembers before that awakening? Needless to say, a corroborative history must be obtained from an observer. If the spouse says he was "talking crazy," one searches for the details, keeping in mind what one would have examined if present. Perhaps he was talking about the recently deceased as though they were still alive—evidence for retrograde amnesia. Perhaps he repeated the same question many times, even a simple question like "what is for dinner?"—evidence for an inability to form new memories. Figure 1 summarizes the clinical picture of the amnestic syndrome, particularly as related to trauma.

Differentiation of the amnestic syndrome from other memory complaints is usually not difficult. Many people complain of slight difficulties in remembering things. This is completely different from a complete memory loss. The clinician should keep in mind four things about generalized mild memory difficulties. First, this may be the initial appearance of dementia. Second, it may represent a symptom of depression. Third, some degree of forgetfulness is normal and need not trigger any further investigation. I have forgotten the fourth thing.

Circumscribed forms of memory loss can be symptoms of focal brain disease. Difficulty in remembering the names of objects forms a major symptom of left-hemisphere dysfunction. Right-hemisphere disease results in a poor memory for faces, maps, and other spatial representations. Chapters 9 and 10 examine these syndromes.

It has been known for centuries that people tend to forget what they do not wish to remember. When gathering material for his theory of evolution, Darwin noted that he could easily remember a fact which agreed with his theory as then formulated, but he had to write down an item which appeared

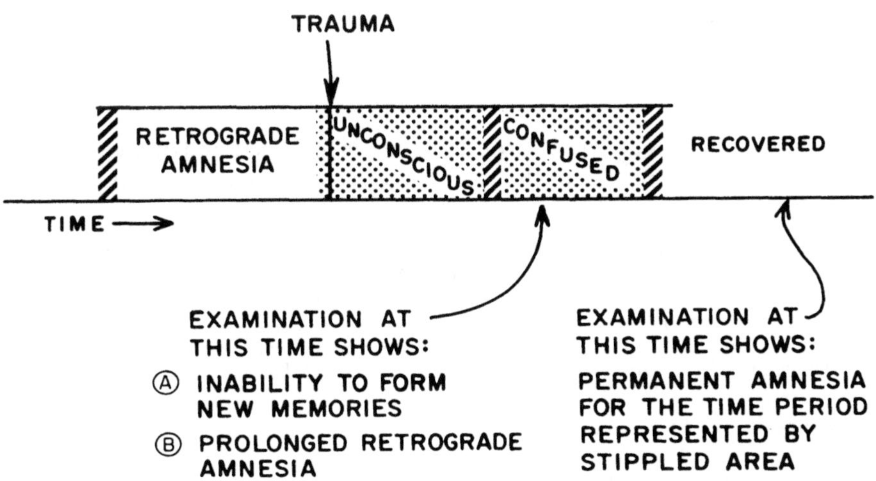

Figure 1: During the period of transient limbic dysfunction following closed head trauma, the patient makes no new memories (cannot place new material in memory stores) and cannot recall the preceding weeks, months, or years (cannot retrieve material from memory). Following limbic reconstitution, the patient can recall events almost, but not quite up to the moment of trauma, but is blank for events that occurred during the period of limbic dysfunction (since this material was never filed).

contrary to his theory or it would soon fade from his memory. Freud institutionalized concepts of repression of emotionally unpleasant memories. The neurologist usually uses the vague and undefinable adjective "hysterical" for any type of amnesia not associated with brain dysfunction. The psychiatrist tries to separate unconsciously repressed elements from consciously feigned amnesia. The patient with feigned amnesia may not know who he is—unlike the truly amnestic. The malingering amnestic has the vocabulary of a high school or college graduate, yet he can not recall such grade school facts as the first President or the nation's capital.

ETIOLOGIC DIAGNOSIS

If the patient describes one or more amnestic spells but his current examination results are normal, etiologic considerations are restricted to a limited number of specific entities. These include seizures, ischemia, certain drug intoxications, and the condition termed transient global amnesia. A consecutive series of patients, referred to a neurological center, is presented in Table 1. While transient global amnesia was the most common diagnosis in this center, one might expect different results in a primary practice or a center with a smaller referral pattern.

Seizures

Epileptic seizures generally produce amnesia for the period of unconsciousness, but only rarely cause the true amnestic syndrome. Nevertheless, the

TABLE 1: Consecutive Patients Referred to a Neurological Center for Evaluation of Transient Amnesia

Final Diagnosis	*Cases*	*Percentage*
Transient global amnesia (single episode)	15	39
Amnesia due to transient ischemia	9	23
Amnesia due to psychomotor seizures	7	18
Amnesia associated with migraine attacks	2	5
Amnesia following encephalitis	2	5
Psychogenic or feigned amnesia	4	10

(Croft et al., 1973, with a subset reported in greater detail by Heathfield et al., 1973)

sudden onset and subsequent confusion can produce a frightening memory loss, as in this patient's description of his first major motor seizure:

> I was watching television when I fell asleep, I guess. When I woke up I was sore all over. I had a bruise on my back, a lump on my head, and cuts here on my tongue. When I looked around I saw plants on the floor, everything messed up. At first I thought there had been an earthquake but there were some areas in my room that weren't affected at all.

The absence attack of petit mal epilepsy usually, but not always, creates a blank in the ongoing stream of consciousness. Videotape studies show that memory remains normal for the first two or three seconds of the EEG spike-wave discharge in most petit mal attacks; in a few, however, the seizure produces a retrograde amnesia for the second or two preceding the EEG discharge (Freemon et al., 1972).

The full amnestic syndrome can occur with temporal lobe or psychomotor seizures (Greene and Bennett, 1974; Gilbert, 1978). Since Chapter 11 is devoted to this type of seizure disorder, comments here are restricted to an illustrative case. A 25-year-old married woman was admitted to the hospital for evaluation of psychomotor seizures. The next day, I saw her in the patients' day room looking as though she didn't know where she was. When asked her name, she gave her maiden name; when asked her age she said 18. I was about to test her ongoing memory abilities when she blinked her eyes a few times and asked "What happened?" She knew where she was and her correct name and age, but had no recollection of the preceding minutes.

The memory loss following seizures produced by shock therapy has been studied in great detail. In general, after several induced seizures the amnestic syndrome occurs. Subjects can remember items for up to 24 seconds, but not for 30 seconds (Stones, 1973). Some items seen just before the induced seizure can be recalled eight hours later, but not two hours later (Patterson et al., 1978). During the period of maximum confusion, a retrograde amnesia of many years is apparent (Squire, 1975). Although histopathological changes probably result from repeated shock treatments (Friedberg, 1977), memory testing reverts completely to normal after a short while (Squire and Chace, 1975).

Ischemia

Transient ischemic attacks of the vertebrobasilar system are quite common, but only rarely do these produce the amnestic syndrome. In most, but not all humans, a small branch of the posterior cerebral artery provides blood supply to the hippocampal complex (Muller and Shaw, 1965).

Decreased flow through the vertebrobasilar system might produce bilateral hippocampal ischemia and limbic memory disorder in these individuals.

Diagnosis is based upon repeated, brief episodes of amnesia associated with other symptoms of posterior circulation ischemia. The syndrome has occurred as a complication of cardiac catheterization (Shuttleworth and Wise, 1973). Unlike other forms of the amnestic syndrome, some of the patients with ischemia show neurological abnormalities on examination after memory has returned to normal—neurological abnormalities indicating infarction in the vertebrobasilar arterial territory (Heathfield et al., 1973). Treatment with aspirin or anticoagulation medication should decrease the number of these attacks.

Occasionally, the amnestic syndrome occurs in association with migraine headaches. Diagnosis is based upon associated symptoms such as preceding scintillating scotoma (Gilbert and Benson, 1972). The memory deficit is presumably related to the intracranial vasoconstrictive phase of the migraine attack. Confusional migraine, not uncommon in childhood, represents a more global disorganization of attention and cognition than the amnestic syndrome (Ehyai and Fenichel, 1978).

Drug Induced Amnesia

Certain drugs can produce the transient limbic memory disorder. These include anticholinergic agents in large doses, benzodiazepines, certain general anesthetics, and alcohol. Drug induced anterograde amnesia is often not associated with retrograde amnesia—a phenomenon seen only rarely in other causes of limbic memory disorder (Squire and Slater, 1978). The anticholinergics, especially scopolamine, produce memory loss when intravenously administered in high doses. This effect is readily reversed by physostigmine (Drachman, 1977). The benzodiazepines, especially diazepam, produce a typical anterograde amnesia when injected intravenously (Clark et al., 1979) and occasionally produce amnesia following large oral doses (Gilbert and Benson, 1972). Certain anesthetics, especially ketamine, were specifically developed to produce a dream-like state, wherein a patient could cooperate during minor surgical or diagnostic procedures, yet not remember these events (Pender, 1971). A large number of anesthetics in appropriate doses can also produce ongoing memory deficit. These include the inhalation agents nitrous oxide (Brice et al., 1970) and methoxyflurane (Reier and Hamelberg, 1969), as well as the intravenous agents already mentioned. Mazzia and Randt (1966) observed that amnesia occurred during light inhalation of anesthesia only when the eyes assumed an abnormal posture, each eye drifting laterally into a position of divergent strabismus. A patient has been reported with transient limbic memory disorder, probably due to digitalis intoxication (Greenlee et al., 1975).

The most common drug-induced amnestic state is the alcohol blackout. The person with this is speaking, walking, or driving (hopefully not) as well as anyone who is mildly intoxicated, but later he has no recollection of these acts. This syndrome is represented in television and cinema by the comedian with a hangover, who sheepishly calls his host to ask, "Did I have a good time last night?" Detailed mental status examination of individuals during this state shows an inability to form new memories exactly concomitant in time with the subsequent period of amnesia (Goodwin et al., 1970). Actually, the amnesia is not quite total, since some elements remain at an emotional level; shown a container full of live worms, for example, the subject may not the next day recall the contents of the container, yet he may know it is unpleasant. Some have hypothesized that the alcohol triggered a temporal lobe seizure (Ryback, 1970), but the EEG recorded during the blackout shows only slowing of the background rhythm, a characteristic of alcohol intoxication with or without amnesia (Freemon et al., 1971). Apparently, the alcoholic blackout is as old as alcohol. In the first act of *Othello*, Cassio imbibes too much and later laments, "I remember a mass of things but nothing distinctly; a quarrel, but nothing wherefor. O God, that men should put an enemy in their mouths to steal away their brains!"

Transient Global Amnesia

Some use the term transient global amnesia (TGA) for the clinical syndromes described in this chapter. For example, Gilbert and Benson (1972) report two cases of TGA with definite etiologies, one associated with migraine and the other following the ingestion of 500 mg of diazepam. Most, however, use the term for a single occurrence of the amnestic syndrome lasting for several hours (Bender, 1960; Fisher and Adams, 1964; Shuttleworth and Morris, 1966; Erkulvrawatr et al., 1979). This very day a medical student related to me a harrowing experience which probably represents an occurrence of TGA. As he and his grandfather were leaving a restaurant and about to get into the latter's car, the grandfather stepped back and asked, "Whose car is this?" He then spontaneously asked the student their location. The student informed him, but after the passage of just a few minutes the question was asked again. The grandfather's repeated questions frightened the student, who is only a sophomore, and he performed a rudimentary examination including a normal blood pressure. Three hours later, when the student found a physician, the grandfather's memory was normal except that he could not remember anything that had occurred since lunch.

Some consider this entity—transient global amnesia—to be a seizure (Gilbert, 1978), but normal EEGs have been recorded even during the period of ongoing memory deficit (Jaffe and Bender, 1966). Many are convinced that this entity is a transient ischemic attack. Nausieda and Sherman (1979), for example, actually begin their report with the declaration that "transient global amnesia is generally believed to be a transient ischemic attack affecting short-term memory centers." The typical attack, however, is much longer than most TIAs, and in the vast majority of cases TGA consists of a single episode. I think it best to consider this entity idiopathic (but organic) amnesia. If one insists on a working model or hypothesis, one can think of transient global amnesia as an infarction of one hippocampus, associated with transient dysfunction of the other by the series of mechanisms described in Chapter 2 under the rubric of diaschisis. Lisak and Zimmerman (1977) reported a patient with transient global amnesia and a malignant tumor of the left hemisphere, probably a coincidental association.

PERMANENT MEMORY LOSS

Temporary dysfunction of certain portions of the limbic system produces the amnestic syndrome described in this chapter. Destruction of these same areas causes a permanent, ongoing memory deficit. Three disease entities produce the vast majority of permanent memory disorder; bilateral hippocampal infarction, herpes simplex encephalitis, and Korsakov's disease. Certain other entities should be mentioned also. Occasionally, closed-head trauma is so severe that whatever process underlies the facile term reconstitution of memory function cannot overcome the degree of brain damage. The longest known duration of anterograde amnesia before recovery is eight years; this record belongs to Mr. Gene Tipps of Texas. A very rare case of penetrating brain injury may cause the amnestic syndrome. Jarho (1973) found 11 such cases in 1556 soliders wounded in the Finnish wars against the Soviet Union; these 11 individuals had a wound tract which crossed the midline in the thalamic region. Very rarely, a patient with a midline brain tumor exhibits predominant memory symptoms (Sprofkin and Sciarra, 1952; Heilman and Sypert, 1977; Ziegler et al., 1977). One patient with prolonged limbic memory disorder improved following drainage of a cystic craniopharyngioma (Ignelzi and Squire, 1976), and another with variable memory loss improved following surgical removal and radiotherapy of the large chromophobe adenoma (Hartley et al., 1974). Permanent limbic memory dysfunction can very rarely follow subarachnoid hemorrhage (Theander and Granholm, 1967). Certain rare degenerative diseases can result in ongoing memory loss (Newton et al., 1971). Partial degeneration of limbic structures can produce a weakening of memory without true amnesia (a clinical picture of dementia), especially the central or axial form of dementia, considered in the next chapter.

Bilateral Hippocampal Infarction

We have already discussed the variable blood supply to hippocampal structures and how transient decreased blood flow through the vertebrobasilar system can, in some individuals, produce a transient ischemic attack characterized by amnesia. This ischemia, if prolonged, can lead to infarction. The unfortunate victim of this bilateral stroke looks alert and has no paralysis, but has a permanent retrograde amnesia for 10 or more years and a total inability to form new memories. Cases studied clinically and at postmortem have been reported by Victor et al. (1961) and by DeJong (1973). Very rarely, a transient amnestic syndrome, perhaps lasting several months, can follow unilateral (left) hippocampal infarction (Mohr et al., 1971; Benson et al., 1974). Limbic memory loss can also occur with bilateral infarction of the medial thalamus; some of these patients have an associated loss of voluntary vertical eye movements (Mills and Swanson, 1978).

Often, decreased flow through the basilar artery produces bilateral occipital infarction and cortical blindness. A rare individual with cortical blindness may have associated memory loss, probably representing combined bilateral occipital and hippocampal infarction. These patients have a complete disregard of the blindness and even claim to be able to see normally. This syndrome is named after Anton. Although no cases have come to autopsy and few have had their memory disorder clearly defined, Anton's syndrome, in most instances, probably represents the permanent limbic memory disorder (Sugar and Goldstein, 1965).

Herpes Simplex Encephalitis

For unclear reasons, the herpes simplex virus preferentially attacks the orbitofrontal and temporal neocortices and the hippocampal complex. The initial clinical picture is delirium, but as neuronal death follows neuronal irritation, the memory disorder supervenes. At this point, the pneumoencephalogram shows hippocampal atrophy reflected by dilatation of the temporal horns of the lateral ventricles (Muramoto et al., 1979). Antiviral therapy early in the course of the disease decreases mortality (Whitley et al., 1977); by the time memory disorder is apparent, however, such therapy is useless.

Other forms of inflammation restricted to the temporal lobes have been described (Friedman and Allen, 1969). Some of these probably represent instances of undiagnosed herpes simplex encephalitis. Some patients who also have cancer have been reported (Corsellis et al., 1968); this paraneoplastic syndrome may result from abnormal immune defenses.

Korsakov's Disease

Korsakov's disease is due to thiamine deficiency. In Western civilization, chronic alcoholism almost always underlies the dietary deficiency, but the disorder has occurred in a wide variety of medical and sociological circumstances, including prisoner-of-war camps (Smith, 1946; Denny-Brown, 1947). Thiamine deficiency also produces a sensorimotor polyneuropathy, so that most patients with newly diagnosed Korsakov's disease have absent ankle jerks, weakness of distal muscle, and a sensory loss in a stocking-glove distribution.

As thiamine pyrophosphate, thiamine or vitamin B_1 serves as a co-factor in a large number of enzymatic reactions, particularly in the glycolytic pathway and the citric-acid cycle. Since ethanol is metabolized via acetaldehyde to acetate, which enters the citric-acid cycle, persons who obtain most of their calories from alcohol are particularly susceptible to thiamine deficiency. The peripheral neuropathy of thiamine deficiency often begins with bilateral foot drop. Sensory symptoms are present, but in thiamine deficiency pain is usually not prominent. The peripheral neuropathy can be present alone, or can be associated with Korsakov's disease or with cardiac failure. Why thiamine deficiency strikes some patients with a peripheral neuropathy, some with Korsakov's disorder, some with heart failure, and others with a combination of these syndromes cannot be explained. Perhaps environmental factors such as the level of dietary constituents other than thiamine determine which of these disorders will develop first. Blass and Gibson (1977) found decreased binding of thiamine pyrophosphate to the enzyme transketolase in patients with the Wernicke-Korsakov syndrome.

Some feel that Korsakov's disease always presents with Wernicke's encephalopathy, but the lifestyle of some alcoholics does not permit detailed evaluation of symptom progression in all cases. Wernicke's encephalopathy is the acute onset of a global depression of attention and cognition with ataxia and abnormal eye movements, especially nystagmus. Some of the most florrid cases have an associated hypothermia (Lipton et al., 1978). As the gross mental dysfunction of the Wernicke syndrome disappears, the memory deficit of Korsakov's disease becomes apparent. Most Korsakov patients have a retrograde amnesia of at least 20 years (Albert et al., 1979). Treatment with thiamine early in the progression of these symptoms can produce significant memory improvement (Victor et al., 1971). It is important to give the thiamine intravenously because alcoholics (perhaps because of chronic alcoholic gastritis) absorb thiamine poorly (Thomson et al., 1970).

The underlying pathology in Korsakov's disease was until recently thought to involve mammillary bodies. These nuclei are important way stations in the posterior hypothalamus, receiving input from the fornix and sending output to the anterior thalamic nucleus. Careful review of their clinical and autopsy findings convinced Victor, Adams, and Collins (1971) that the memory loss correlated best with neuronal dropout in the dorsomedial thalamic nucleus—part of the limbic thalamus which projects to orbitofrontal cortex. Grunnet (1969) has found a change in the histopathology of Wernicke's disease since the introduction of thiamine therapy. Noradrenergic portions of the brain are probably involved, since Korsakov patients have decreased noradrenergic metabolites in the CSF (McEntree and Mair, 1978).

As an aside, we should repeat that a few clinicians use the term Korsakov's disease for any patient with the amnestic syndrome, regardless of etiology. The term should probably be restricted to those patients with ongoing memory deficit secondary to thiamine deficiency.

Confabulation and Other Symptoms

While the memory disorder forms the most outstanding feature of patients with bilateral limbic destruction, certain associated symptoms deserve mention. Most of these patients have a bland but pleasant personality; they have little concern or affect. A few have mild sexual aberrations; the male patient reported by Terzian and Dalle Ore (1955) showed a pathetic exhibitionism. This constellation of symptoms bears some resemblance to the sexual abnormalities and lack of fear seen in monkeys following bilateral removal of medial temporal structures (Kluver and Bucy, 1939). Some have used the term Kluver-Bucy syndrome to refer to patients with ongoing memory loss and associated hypoemotionality (Pilleri, 1966; Shraberg and Weisberg, 1978). The habit of these monkeys to place unfamiliar objects in their mouths (called visual agnosia by Kluver and Bucy) is not part of the human syndrome.

Many textbooks define confabulation so broadly that it becomes a normal phenomenon. At my high school reunion, for example, a man came up to me, stuck out his hand, and said: "Hi, Frank, remember me, I'm Phil Harrison." He certainly looked familiar so I shook his hand and replied, "Of course I remember you, Phil." No one in our class was named Phil Harrison, and I had been confabulating which I realized when Jimmy Gauger broke into laughter at the joke on his old boyhood chum.

However, pathological confabulation does exist. The patient spontaneously originates imaginative, even wild, stories. The examiner can sometimes trigger these by asking the patient if they have previously met. The normal person may reluctantly admit to a possible interaction in a previous medical setting. The confabulatory individual starts an endless story about his adventures with the examiner. "Sure, I saw you yesterday on Broad Street; you had your spotted dog with you, the one with the diamond collar, and . . ." Pathological confabulation is usually, but not always, a symptom of Korsakov's disease (Mercer et al., 1977). Some have hypothesized that it is a learned behavior associated with many hours of spinning tall tales in the barroom; but most likely, true pathological confabulation in an organic phenomenon. Stuss and co-workers (1978) have presented clinical evidence linking this symptom to a combination of limbic and frontal lobe lesions.

ILLUSTRATIVE CASES

A 49-year-old truck driver developed strange behavior after awakening from a syncopal attack. He wandered about the house, bumping into walls, and became combative when his wife tried to restrain him. He even claimed that she was not his wife. The admitting physician described generalized cerebellar dysfunction and severe memory disorder, but did not recognize that the patient was blind.

When I first saw the patient he was lying in bed with head and eyes turned toward his right, toward the window. He had nystagmus with normally reactive pupils. The patient could repeat six numbers easily.

Examiner: They tell me you are having trouble with your memory.
Patient: A little.
Examiner: Give me an example of how your memory bothers you.
Patient: (Pauses as though thinking but never answers.)
Examiner: How old are you?
Patient: 38 (actually he was 49).
Examiner: What year is this?
Patient: (After a pause) 1970 (actually it was 1973).
Examiner: When is your birthdate?
Patient: (Without hesitation) September 15, 1923.
Examiner: Who is the President?
Patient: Huh?
Examiner: Who is the President of the U.S.A.?
Patient: I never pay attention.
Examiner: Who is the last President that stands out in your mind?
Patient: Truman.
Examiner: Who came after Truman?

Patient: I don't know.

Examiner: Did you ever hear of John F. Kennedy?

Patient: No.

Examiner: What happened to him?

Patient: He was shot.

Examiner: Are you married?

Patient: Yes.

Examiner: How long?

Patient: About 15 years (actually he was divorced and remarried about a year previously).

Examiner: What is this town we are in?

Patient: Chattanooga (actually it was Nashville).

Examiner: How is your vision?

Patient: OK.

Examiner: How many fingers am I holding up? (Five).

Patient (Without hesitation) One.

Examiner: How many now (Two, hand moved).

Patient: One.

Examiner: No, you are looking in the wrong place, over here. (Hand moved up and down; patient looks toward examiner's face but not his hand.)

This patient had had decreased flow through his vertebrobasilar system, giving him cerebellar signs, cortical blindness, and limbic memory disorder. This denial of blindness is an example of Anton's syndrome. He died of heart failure two years later; autopsy could not be obtained.

A 64-year-old left-handed retired male was found unconscious on the floor of his apartment. Upon awakening in the hospital, he had a marked memory deficit. He named the city correctly, but did not know he was in a hospital, one time guessing he was in a barber shop. He gave the year on various examinations as some time in the 1950's or 1960's. He gave Eisenhower as President; he recognized the name Kennedy as President but did not know of the assassination. His memory of his childhood seemed clear although no corroborative source was available. The patient's minister reported that his knowledge of Biblical quotations was better than it had ever been, but he reluctantly acknowledged that the patient did not recognize him as his minister. If the examiner placed a single item in his pocket the patient could name the item after the passage of one minute, but had no idea after the passage of ten minutes. The patient also had cerebellar signs, and a right homonymous hemianopsia. Over the course of two months, some improvement occurred; the patient finally began to recognize his doctors.

The patient died of pneumonia, and autopsy showed an infarction involving the left hippocampal complex (Figure 2).

A 56-year-old housewife had developed severe memory loss after herpes simplex encephalitis, which had occurred two years earlier. She now had a very bland, but pleasant personality, frequently clasping the hand of a nurse spontaneously and saying, "God bless you." She had a severe retrograde memory loss and could not create new memories. The latter was tested by placing a small object under one of three boxes. If the examiner sat with her, reminding her to concentrate on the "shell game" she could, after five minutes elapsed, identify the object under the correct box and describe it in detail. If the examiner engaged her attention in the interim, however, she could specify the correct box, but not its contents, in up to 60 seconds. After the passage of 90 seconds, she forgot the game completely. To test memory for spatial function, the patient was asked to assemble six interlocking jigsaw pieces. Each time she tried this, after several minutes of intervening conversation, the assembly took approximately 30 seconds. If the pieces were undone while she watched, she could reassemble them in five seconds; if she waited several minutes, her performance again deteriorated to the 30 second baseline. Here is a recorded interview:

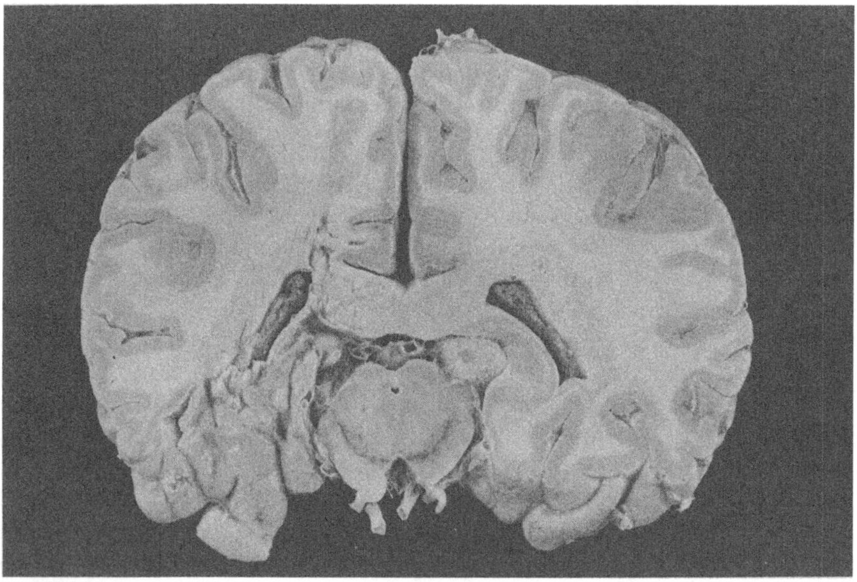

Figure 2: Infarction of the left hippocampal complex produced limbic memory dysfunction in this 64-year-old man. The patient died two months after the stroke. If he had survived would memory have returned to normal?

Examiner: Can you give me an example of how your memory bothers you?

Patient: Well, if my brother came over or something, and he wanted to tell me something, say he was going to come and tell me he was going to visit me again, then I would have to keep asking, well, what day is today, and I said if I had a piece of paper I would write it down. Then I would put the date, what today is, and then if you tell me like, for instance . . . he says he will come about the 12th or something and if today is not the 12th . . . say its the 9th or something then I see I put the date on there. That is the way I would do it.

Examiner: Let's test your memory a little. I'm going to put something in my pocket right here. Do you see what it is?

Patient: Yes, it is a penny.

Examiner: Yes, hold it in your hand a second and you, why don't you yourself drop it in my pocket right here.

Patient: All right.

Examiner: Now, what do I have in my pocket.

Patient: A penny, one penny.

Examiner: Yes, that's right. I'm going to ask that you remember that. I noticed that you are playing solitaire right now (the patient had been playing solitaire and cards were on the desk in front of her).

Patient: Yes.

Examiner: Let's take one of these cards and see if you can remember it. What card is this?

Patient: That's the ace of spades. I can see it.

Examiner: Yes, let me turn it upside down. Now do you recall that I asked you to remember something that I put in my pocket?

Patient: (Looks puzzled.)

Examiner: What do I have in my pocket here? (touching to pocket)

Patient: Nothing.

Examiner: No, look here, I have a penny in my hand, right here and I'm going to put it in my pocket. Now what do I have in my pocket here?

Patient: Now you have a penny.

Examiner: Right. Now what card is this? (pointing to the upside-down ace of spades)

Patient: That's the ace of hearts.

Examiner: No, it is the ace of spades. Let me turn it upside down again, do you know what it is now?

Patient: Yes, it is the ace of spades.

Examiner: And what do I have in my pocket?

Patient: A penny.

Examiner: Right. Now I wonder if you could tell me a little bit about your past life?

Patient: My past life? Well, I worked for the Heil Company for many years, in shorthand and typing. And I played violin in the Young Peoples' Orchestra, too, for many years. I like to play the violin, you know. At Young Peoples', we played everything: classical, modern, even church music.

Examiner: What was the most modern song that you played?

Patient: The most modern, let me see. One of my favorites was Beethoven's Fifth Symphony.

Examiner: Well, that's not too modern. That's not exactly what I had in mind, but let me test your memory again about something else. Do you remember that a while ago I asked you to remember something?

Patient: Yes, about what I did in the past.

Examiner: Well, before that. Did I ask you to remember where I put something?

Patient: No.

Examiner: I put something someplace and I asked you to remember it.

Patient: Something in your pocket?

Examiner: Right, absolutely right. Do you recall what it is?

Patient: No, I don't remember what it is.

Examiner: But you did recall that it is in my pocket?

Patient: Yes, it is in a pocket. It is a . . . (thinking, long pause)

Examiner: Well, it's a penny. Let me show it to you.

Patient: Oh, it's a penny.

Examiner: Do you remember about that card there (pointing to the upside-down card).

Patient: The card? It's a king.

Examiner: No, it's not a king. Why don't you guess again, that's very close.

Patient: Ace.

Examiner: Ace of what?

Patient: Ace of hearts.

Examiner: No, actually it's the ace of spades. Let me show you. That's very close. Let me ask you some other memory questions. Can you name our President? Name a recent President?

Patient: Hoover.

Examiner: Hoover, good. Who was President after Hoover?

Patient: I don't remember who was after Hoover.

Examiner: Who was President during the war?

Patient: I was thinking of Roosevelt.

Examiner: Roosevelt, absolutely right. Can you recall anyone after Roosevelt?

Patient: No.

Examiner: If I were to give you three names, do you think you could pick the right guy out of those three names?

Patient: Let's see.

Examiner: How about these three names: Williams, Truman, Henderson.

Patient: Truman, yeah. I remember Truman.

Examiner: Who came after Truman, can you recall?

Patient: No, I don't remember who came after him.

Examiner: Let me give you three names and see if you can recall which one of these he was. He was a general in the war. Try these names. Roba, Eisenhower, and Trimensky.

Patient: Eisenhower, yes.

Examiner: I bet you can't name who came after Eisenhower, though?

Patient: No, I don't remember.

Examiner: It was Kennedy. Do you remember what happened to Kennedy?

Patient: No, I don't.

Examiner: He died.

Patient: He wasn't killed, he just died from illness?

Examiner: Yes, he actually was killed. Do you remember that?

Patient: He was killed? No, somebody might have said that, that's why it came to my mind about the killing.

Examiner: Can you name the approximate year this year?

Patient: 1965 (actually it was 1971).

Examiner: Do you remember the day you were born.

Patient: June 9, 1915.

Examiner: Do you remember the day you were married?

Patient: No, I don't remember the day I was married.

Examiner: But you were married?

Patient: Yes, I was, but I don't remember how old I was though.

Examiner: Do you remember your childhood very well?

Patient: You mean when I was a young kid? Like I said, I lived at 1906 West Driman Avenue and I worked at the Heil Company and played violin in the Young Peoples' Symphony Orchestra.

Examiner: How old were you then?

Patient: When I played the violin I must have been 18 or 19.

Examiner: I wonder if you can guess what card this might be right here that is upside down.

Patient: It's a jack.

Examiner: No, it's not a jack.

Patient: It's a joker?

Examiner: No, it's not a joker. We actually took the joker out.

Patient: Is it an ace?

Examiner: Absolutely right, it's an ace. It's an ace of what?

Patient: Hearts?

Examiner: You keep guessing hearts, but actually the card is a spade (turning card upright).

Patient: Spades.

Examiner: You must have hearts on your mind. A little while ago I put something someplace and asked you to remember what it was.

Patient: Where my bed is?

Examiner: I know you know how to find your bed, because you asked the nurses to put your name on it. Do you remember that?

Patient: Just like that, with my name on it?

Examiner: Do you know the name of this building that we are in now? Sometimes you have told me correctly.

Patient: Young Peoples' General Hospital is what I was thinking of.

Examiner: I wonder if you could tell me about how old you are, approximately?

Patient: Approximately 41 or 42.

Examiner: This year is actually 1971, so how old are you?

Patient: 56. Oh, yes, past my middle age.

Chapter 8

Dementia

CLINICAL PRESENTATION

The syndrome of dementia is characterized by progressive chronic deterioration of intellectual function. The term dementia implies organic dysfunction of brain cells producing poor memory; impaired judgement; decreased attention; and loss of arithmetic, reasoning, and problem-solving abilities. Some use the term presenile dementia to refer to any dementing process beginning before age 65; others restrict the term to a specific illness—Alzheimer's disease. Since the term presenile has various meanings for different people, and because age 65 has no biological significance, we will not use it.

As in all organic mental diseases, the early clinical picture of dementia varies greatly from one patient to another, depending partly on premorbid personality and partly upon lifestyle. Individuals with a highly demanding, technical career often begin to make a greater frequency of minor errors. They may notice this themselves, or their fellow workers may first observe this slippage. In individuals with more routine work, the initial symptomatology of dementia may involve home activities. Often a relative who visits only occasionally sees a change in the patient-to-be—a change of such insidious onset it has escaped notice by closer relatives. Sometimes the type of change cannot be specified in detail, even in retrospect; the patient just isn't himself.

The initial symptom may involve memory. The patient has the same memory foibles he has always had, but now they are more frequent and more noticeable. He must look up telephone numbers twice or ask his spouse where things are placed. As the disease progresses, most patients develop some degree of depression, reacting to their recognition of their decreasing intellectual powers (Liston, 1977). As the mental deterioration worsens, neurological abnormalities sometimes appear. These findings—generally referred to as "frontal lobe" signs—include the palmomental and snout reflexes (Paulson and Gottlieb, 1968). Not all patients, however, develop these signs even with advanced dementia, and they are sometimes present in normal subjects; therefore, these findings must be interpreted in the context of the full clinical picture.

Some physicians have attempted to differentiate two presentations of the dementia syndrome. In one of these dementia subtypes, the major clinical symptom is apathy and withdrawal. The patient appears abnormal even to a superficial observer. He does not speak unless spoken to. He often shows a drab and lifeless facial expression, punctuated by episodes of uncontrollable sobbing. The "frontal lobe" signs previously mentioned may be present on neurological examination. In the other form of dementia, the major symptom is memory loss. To a nonmedical observer, the patient appears normal. He has what has been termed a "cocktail party" personality; superficial discussion of general topics are normal, but deeper investigation reveals enormous memory holes. The patient may engage in a lively repartee on the lack of morals or intelligence of governmental leaders, but when questioned on specifics it becomes apparent he does not even know the name of the President. Some experts have attempted to differentiate the latter memory disorder—referred to as limbic or subcortical dementia—from the more global deficit of the previously described "frontal lobe" or cortical dementia. While extremes are easily differentiated, most patients fall between the two. Some degenerative disorders, especially Alzheimer's disease, show a progression; the early case is more "limbic," the deteriorated patient more "cortical."

SYNDROME DIAGNOSIS

The patient suffering from dementia must be differentiated from patients suffering from other conditions which masquerade as a progressive decline in intellectual function. Many dementia patients suffer a reactive depression usually early in the course of the development of the dementia (Liston, 1977). Because of this, one cannot really separate depression from dementia but rather, one evaluates depressed patients to see if there is any underlying component of dementia. Midlife depression is a common problem; these patients commonly complain of memory difficulty (Kahn et al., 1975). Often there is extensive psychomotor retardation, and examination of these patients can be very tiring. If the patient is depressed but not demented, great patience on the part of the examiner will slowly disclose answers that are normal in content. Normal neuropsychological testing in the depressed patient is often valuable in determining that no underlying dementia is present; abnormal test results are less valuable. In the final analysis, it is sometimes necessary to treat depression by pharmacological means and await a clinical response (Shraberg, 1978). The depression may clear completely and the patient return to normal; in other patients the depression will lift and dementia will be clearly seen. Clinical differentiation of dementia from depression and other psychiatric syndromes has been reviewed by Wells (1979).

Another common differential diagnosis concerns dementia versus aphasia. While most patients with aphasia have associated symptoms of left-hemispheral dysfunction such as right hemiparesis or hemianopsia, there are some patients who have parietal lesions that produce a predominantly sensory or Wernicke aphasia with few other signs. These individuals have great difficulty in understanding speech as well as in reading. They have difficulty following an examiner's line of questioning, and superficial evaluation may lead the physician to suspect dementia. A more detailed mental status examination usually quickly identifies a patient who has aphasic symptomatology such as inability to name common objects. The aphasia is usually due to a vascular problem, often an embolus, and is of sudden onset while the dementia syndrome is insidiously progressive.

ETIOLOGIC DIAGNOSIS

Potentially Reversible Causes

Once he determines that a patient suffers the syndrome of dementia, the physician looks for the underlying cause. Many degenerative brain diseases produce dementia. These disorders, diagnosed by histological examination of brain tissue, are designated by a series of eponyms: Alzheimer, Binswanger, Pick, Kraeplin, Behcet, Hallevorden-Spatz. Academic neurologists love to argue about the best eponym to apply to a given clinical picture but this diagnosis has limited practical value.

In my opinion, the diagnostic effort in etiologic diagnoses should be directed toward the identification of treatable illnesses. A large number of medical and neurological diseases at least partially reversible by appropriate specific therapy can present as dementia. Several other disorders amenable to specific therapy include mental changes as part of their symptomatology, but the clinical picture of dementia does not predominate (see Chapter 6). Wilson's disease can present as personality change or even psychosis; Kayser-Fleischer rings will be present at that point in the development of the disease. Similarly, porphyria can produce striking mental changes, such as vivid hallucinations, but is never really associated with the full dementia syndrome. Although most patients with Parkinson's disease are mentally normal, some have an associated dementia; in all these patients, treatment is aimed at countering the motor manifestations of parkinsonism while no specific therapy counters the cognitive deficits.

Table 1 summarizes several treatable diseases which can present with progressive intellectual deterioration. Hepatic and renal failure frequently produce dementia; usually, but not always, however, other symptoms and signs make diagnosis obvious. Hypothyroidism frequently presents with slowed thinking; diagnosis can be especially difficult in elderly individuals with atrophic skin and absent ankle reflexes (Morrow, 1978). Dementia, weight loss, and proximal muscle weakness occur with hyperthyroidism in the elderly, but the absence of tachycardia and enlargement of the thyroid gland can make diagnosis difficult (Thomas et al., 1970). Neurosyphilis can cause dementia with or without associated neurological findings such as irregular pupils and areflexia. Mental improvement, but not normalization, can be expected following high dosage penicillin therapy. Mental improvement occurred with arsenical treatment of tertiary syphilis in the preantibiotic era (Matthews et al., 1938). High levels of circulating lipids can produce intellectual deterioration (Heilman and Fisher, 1974), as can frequent petit mal or temporal lobe seizures (Doose and Volzke, 1979).

Certain vitamin deficiencies also produce dementia. In 1912, 10,000 hospital beds in the United States were occupied by demented patients suffering from pellagra. The recognition by the infectious-disease expert

TABLE 1: Remedial Causes of Dementia

Normal pressure hydrocephalus (Hakim-Adams syndrome)

Chronic drug intoxication

Mass lesions
  a. frontal lobe tumors
  b. subdural hematomas

Fungal meningitis

Hypothyroidism

Vitamin deficiency
  a. vitamin B_{12} malabsorption
  b. folic acid deficiency
  c. pellagra

Tertiary syphilis

Liver or renal failure

Temporal lobe or psychomotor seizure status

Joseph Goldberger that this entity was a deficiency disease, the subsequent identification of the vitamin niacin, and the virtual elimination of the disorder by the fortification of bread, is one of the great triumphs of medical science in this century (reviewed by Barrett-Connor, 1967). Pellagra is still occasionally seen in the most severe alcoholics.

Thiamine deficiency can produce Korsakov's disease. The severe memory loss, coupled with preservation of other cognitive functions, leads most clinicians to classify this disorder as an amnestic syndrome rather than a dementia, as discussed in Chapter 7.

Unlike other deficiency states, vitamin B_{12} deficiency results from malabsorption rather than from an inadequate diet. B_{12} combines in the stomach with an intrinsic factor, a polypeptide secreted by gastric mucosal parietal cells. The B_{12}-intrinsic factor molecule is absorbed in the terminal ileum. Malabsorption can result from a deficiency of the intrinsic factor, from partial gastrectomy (Williams et al., 1969), by destruction of the complex during its traverse of the small intestine, or by malabsorption of the complex because of regional or terminal ileitis. The deficiency state often produces a macrocytic anemia and gastrointestinal symptoms such as sore tongue and poor appetite. The cells of the intestinal mucosa are hypertrophic with small nuclei (Foroozan and Trier, 1967).

The neurological symptoms result from degeneration of oligodendroglial cells in the central nervous system and Schwann cells in the peripheral nervous system with demyelination (Victor and Lear, 1956). Neurological syndromes include optic atrophy, peripheral neuropathy, and subacute degeneration of the spinal cord. Some of the early descriptions of mental changes emphasized persecutory delusions with mild dementia (Herman et al., 1937; Ferraro et al., 1945). Most patients with dementia due to vitamin B_{12} deficiency have an associated macrocytosis, but not an anemia (Roos and Willanger, 1977). Vitamin B_{12} therapy produces significant improvement, usually normalization, of cognitive function (Shulman, 1967).

Until recently, most authorities felt that folic acid deficiency could produce a megaloblastic anemia but not neurological dysfunction. Actually, early studies of experimental folate deficiency in volunteers included symptoms of forgetfulness, remitting with folate therapy (Hebert, 1962). When patients with low folate levels are clinically evaluated, about 70 percent are found to be mildly demented (Reynolds et al., 1973). Severe, long-standing folate deficiency can probably produce cortical atrophy (Botez et al., 1977).

Chronic intoxication with certain drugs leads to progressive intellectual deterioration. For example, the anticonvulsant phenytoin taken for a prolonged period in excessive dosage can produce a clinical picture of dementia (Vallarta et al., 1974). This can occur in cardiac patients as well as in epileptics (Todd and Wilderson, 1978), and may result from interference with folate metabolism (Neubauer, 1970). Dementia can follow chronic use of bromide, still present in a few nonprescription "tonics" (Tylden, 1971). Bromism has also followed industrial pollution of well water (Brenner, 1978). The traditional laxative mercurous chloride, or calomel, may produce mercurialism with dementia (Davis et al., 1974). Other single drug entities reported to cause reversible dementia include methyldopa (Thornton, 1976), quinidine (Gilbert, 1977), and methotrexate (Pizzo et al., 1976). Phenacetin may produce dementia following long-term use, in addition to its well-known renal toxicity (Murray et al., 1971).

Dementia following the prolonged use of several drugs taken simultaneously is more common than dementia produced by a single drug (Maruta, 1978). In a series of 60 consecutive demented patients, five had all mental symptoms resulting from a mixture of depressant drugs such as analgesics, hypnotics, and anticonvulsants. Characteristically, the patients had seen several different practitioners for the same complaint; each physician had prescribed symptomatic treatment. The patients, believing that their doctors' medications, like their knowledge, might have an additive effect, took all of the drugs in the prescribed doses. When these drugs were discontinued or adjusted to more appropriate blood levels, mental function in each of these five patients completely returned to normal (Freemon, 1976).

A few toxins can produce mental deterioration with chronic exposure. Most notable are the heavy metals. The clinician should be especially alert for lead encephalopathy in moonshine drinkers (Asokan et al., 1974) and for mercurialism in dental workers (Smith, 1978). Manganese toxicity has been reported to cause dementia; exposure (except in manganese miners) is from an unknown source, perhaps obsessive abuse of vitamin and mineral supplements (Banta and Markesbery, 1977). Anoxia associated with carbon monoxide posioning can produce a chronic dementing illness which has the appearance of progression (Smith and Brandon, 1973).

The most common treatable causes of progressive intellectual deterioration are depression (considered under the heading *Syndrome Diagnosis*), chronic intoxication of certain depressant drugs (just discussed), mass lesions, and normal pressure hydrocephalus. Mass lesions potentially amenable to therapy include subdural hematomas—particularly bilateral subdural hematomas in the alcoholic, and benign neoplasms—especially parasagittal meningiomas (Hunter et al., 1968). Normal pressure hydrocephalus is such a common, yet such a confusing condition, that it deserves a separate section of this chapter.

Normal Pressure Hydrocephalus

Normal pressure hydrocephalus (NPH) is a poorly understood form of dementia associated with ventricular enlargement. The pathophysiology of this entity remains obscure despite numerous well-described theories; controversy surrounds attempts to delineate diagnostic criteria. It is unquestionable, however, that some patients with the appropriate clinical and radiological picture will improve when CSF is shunted from the lateral ventricle of the brain to the general circulation. Disagreement involves what percentage of patients, how defined, will improve, by how much.

The typical patient presents with dementia, abnormal gait, and frontal lobe signs. The gait is slightly wide based, but not reeling. Difficulty initiating gait (taking the first step) can sometimes appear almost parkinsonoid (Sypert et al., 1973; Mazza et al., 1976). An occasional patient can appear uncooperative and aggressive (Crowell et al., 1973), but apathy and depression are probably more common. The untreated case can progress to the state of akinetic mutism (Moore, 1969). Some clinicians have suggested that the earliest case is represented by mild headaches, forgetfulness, insomnia, and drop attacks (Rice and Gendelman, 1973; Botez et al., 1977). While urinary incontinence is the third item of the so-called characteristic triad of dementia, gait disturbance, and incontinence, it often occurs late in the development of the syndrome and its absence should not deter diagnosis. This symptom sometimes results from lack of social awareness.

Radiological evaluation shows enlarged lateral ventricles with little or no cortical atrophy. Air injected into the lumbar subarachnoid space rises to fill the ventricles, but does not pass over the cerebral convexities (Marions and Lying-Tunell, 1977). In many patients, progressive ventricular dilatation and clinical deterioration occur following pneumoencephalography if the shunt procedure is not performed promptly (Rovit et al., 1972). Computed tomography scanning has largely replaced pneumoencephalography for evaluation of suspected normal pressure hydrocephalus. The flow of air through CSF spaces adds a physiological dimension to pneumoencephalography which is missing from the purely anatomic evaluation of the standard CT scan. Sequential CT scanning to evaluate CSF flow can be performed following the injection of a radio-opaque substance such as metrizamide into lumbar subarachnoid space (Ostertag and Mundinger, 1978).

A similar diagnostic study using radioisotopes is termed cisternography (formerly called RISA-scanning, after the original radioactive material). The isotope passes too slowly over the cerebral convexities of patients with shunt-responsive dementia (Alker et al., 1972) and experimental animals who have developed hydrocephalus after the intrathecal injection of a sclerosing agent (Flor et al., 1974).

Other diagnostic tests have been suggested, but remain in the developmental stage. A series of tests involve measurement of CSF pressure at specified times following the injection of specified volumes of saline into the lumbar subarachnoid space; presumably the NPH patient will have a more rapid rise of pressure because of a block of CSF absorption (Wolinsky et al., 1973;

Trotter et al., 1974; Hartmann and Alberti, 1977). In patients with long standing NPH, the EEG is normal (Brown and Goldensohn, 1973); bursts of rhythmic slow waves occur in some patients, especially those whose dementia responds to shunting (Hashi et al., 1976).

Most theories of pathogenesis assume some sort of block of CSF absorption. The syndrome of NPH can follow meningitis and subarachnoid hemorrhage, conditions which might be expected to produce adhesions in the region of the Pacchionian granules. Most cases with the characteristic clinical and radiological findings, however, have no obvious antecedent cause; this has been called idiopathic NPH, or occult hydrocephalus. Autopsied patients with idiopathic NPH have shown leptomeningeal fibrosis (DeLand et al., 1973; DiRocco et al., 1977). So why isn't the CSF pressure elevated when measured by lumbar puncture? Hakim and Adams (1965) hypothesize that a certain force of pressure is required to push CSF through the absorption mechanism; since force equals pressure times area, a force elevated by meningeal fibrosis could be balanced by an increased area of ventricular wall. Others suggest that NPH is associated with transient or episodic elevations of CSF pressure (Syman et al., 1972); a few patients with the clinical characteristics of NPH, but with chronic pressure elevations, have been reported (Sjaastad and Nornes, 1976). Hoff and Barber (1974) suggest that the pressure gradient between subdural and intraventricular spaces is elevated even when lumbar CSF pressure is not.

It is difficult to determine which patients will improve following the neurosurgical shunt procedure. Some have reported that about one in five demented patients improve regardless of clinical or radiological findings (Salmon, 1972), but most centers report success rates of about 50 percent for patients with apathetic dementia, wide based gait, and enlarged ventricles without cerebral atrophy (see Table 2). Those patients with an identifiable cause have an even greater likelihood of significant improvement. Diagnosis and management fuse; the problem is not one of labelling but, rather, of constructing a cost-benefit ratio. In the words of Messert and Wannamaker (1974):

> the problem does not seem to be merely one of simple diagnosis of whether a patient does or does not have some form of obstructive hydrocephalus, but rather one of determining whether reasonable expectancy of improvement justifies the risks involved in a shunt ing procedure.

The series reviewed in Table 2 show several interesting facts. Those patients who have a demonstrable cause for their hydrocephalus have a greater likelihood of improvement. These causes include disorders which block the flow of CSF from third to fourth ventricles, disorders such as acqueductal stenosis (Murphy et al., 1978), neoplasm including large

TABLE 2: Normal Pressure Hydrocephalus, Results of Shunting

Series	*Diagnostic Criteria*	*Hydrocephalus Etiology*	*Patients Improved After Shunting*
Summary of published series	Full	Occult	85%
(Messert and Wannamaker, 1974)	Incomplete	Occult	50%
Mayo Clinic, Rochester	Full	Occult	74%
(Laws and Mokri, 1977)	Incomplete	Occult	38%
University Hospital, Philadelphia	Full	Known	80%
(Stein and Langfitt, 1974)	Full	Occult	24%
Rikshospitalet, Oslo	Full	Known	59%
(Magnaes, 1978)	Full	Occult	33%

(Occult hydrocephalus means no etiology can be uncovered.)

pituitary adenoma (Shenkin and Crowley, 1973), and an elongated basilar artery (Tonali et al., 1973), as well as causes such as subarachnoid hemorrhage or meningitis which lead to a blockage of CSF absorption over the cerebral convexities (Heck et al., 1971). Secondly, those patients with typical clinical characteristics have a greater chance of mental improvement following shunting than do those patients with atypical features. Detailed analyses of improvement after shunting have shown the presence of gait abnormality and apathetic inertia to be the best predictors (Jacobs et al., 1976; Gustafson and Hagberg, 1978). While the final decision on shunt placement is a surgical one, the general clinician should have enough knowledge of surgical complications to form an opinion. The most common immediate complication is shunt malfunction, occurring in up to 40 percent of patients (Illingsworth et al., 1971). Other immediate complications include subdural and extradural hematomas, and meningitis. A large number of shunted patients, over half in some series, eventually develop epileptic seizures (Ines and Markand, 1977).

Alzheimer's Disease and Senile Dementia

Alzheimer's disease is a slowly dementing disorder associated with intraneuronal neurofibrillary tangles and argyrophilic plaques spread throughout the cerebral cortex. While neurofibrillary tangles occur in many other hereditary and acquired progressive neurological disorders, their distribution and large number characterize Alzheimer's disease (Wisniewski et al., 1979). The tangle probably represents twisted, abnormal neurotubules (Grundke-Iqbal et al., 1979). Neuronal death is followed by cortical atrophy with widened sulci and enlarged ventricles visible on CT scan or pneumoencephalogram. Using grim humor to counter the sadness of this affliction, a neuropathologist has referred to the gross anatomical appearance as "prune brain" (Figure 1).

Although the unequivocal diagnosis requires histological examination of brain tissue, the clinical course is characteristic. Failing memory, associated with neurofibrillary tangles and neuronal dysfunction of the hippocampal complexes, predominates the early phase. More slowly progressive than most other dementias, the pathological process spreads throughout the neocortex. The involvement of the left hemisphere produces decreased verbal output and word searching; right hemisphere cortical dysfunction causes spatial disorientation (getting lost easily). The end stage involves masked facies, increased muscle tone, flexed posture, sometimes myoclonus, and occasionally seizures.

Etiology remains unknown. A small percentage occurs in familial clusters, usually passed by autosomal dominant inheritance (Feldman et al., 1963).

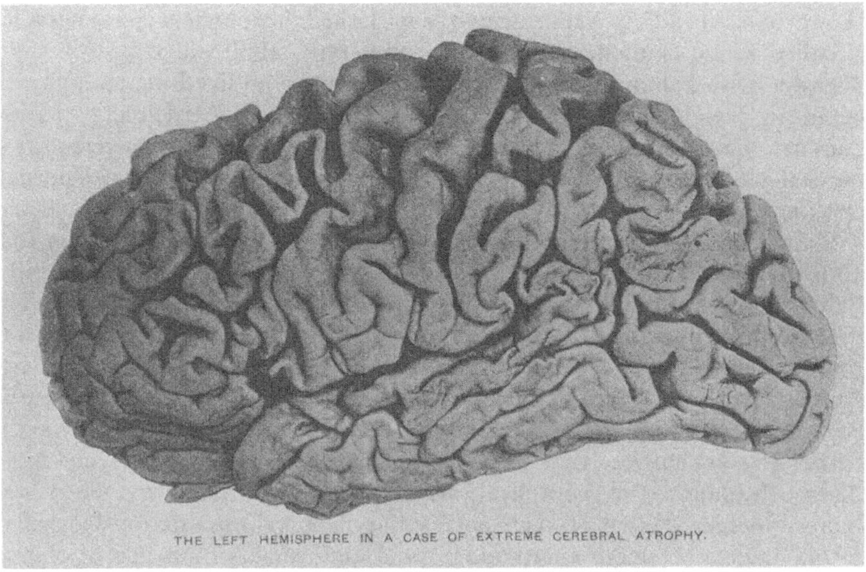

Figure 1: Alzheimer's disease produces severe cortical atrophy. This example is reproduced from Blackburn's (1908) famous insanity atlas.

Some theoreticians have suggested an abnormality somehow related to chromosome 21, since individuals with trisomy 21—Down's syndrome—develop a mental deterioration in their 40s which is clinically and pathologically indistinguishable from Alzheimer's disease (Ellis et al., 1974). Neurofibrillary tangles can be produced in experimental animals by several maneuvers, including administration of aluminum. Elevated tissue levels of aluminum have been found in brains of Alzheimer's disease patients, but the significance of this finding eludes medical science (Trapp et al., 1978). The most promising discovery concerns low activities of the enzyme which synthesizes the neurotransmitter acetylcholine (Davies and Maloney, 1976). This decreased choline acetylase activity does not merely represent general neuronal dropout, since the enzymes of gamma-aminobutyric acid synthesis are normal.

Memory difficulties accelerate with age. The normal aged probably have decreased memory power, so-called benign forgetfulness of senescence. But, in addition, the incidence of true dementia rises dramatically with age. In a few cases, the dementia results from strokes, leading the father of clinical neurology, Jean-Martin Charcot, to declare, "a man is as old as his arteries." Autopsy studies have shown that the predominant histological basis of senile dementia is cortical atrophy with neurofibrillary tangles and argyrophylic plaques, indistinguishable from Alzheimer's disease beginning in middle age

(Todorov et al., 1975). Senile dementia with these histological characteristics is called senile dementia of the Alzheimer type, abbreviated SDAT. This disorder is so common, that perhaps all people who live long enough will begin to feel its effects. Patients with SDAT, like Alzheimer's disease patients, have decreased activity of acetylcholine synthesis in neocortex; normal elderly and those demented from multiple infarcts have normal choline acetylase activity (White et al., 1977).

Senile dementia represents a significant national economic burden that adds to its cost in human misery. Terry (1978) estimates that about one and a half million Americans suffer from some degree of senile dementia. The disorder is responsible for approximately half the elderly patients in nursing homes, representing an annual cost of about six billion dollars. Several studies show an accelerated mortality for individuals with this disease entity (Go et al., 1978). Study of the special fatal risk factors of senile dementia forces the conclusion that these patients die from the underlying brain disease leading to the complications of prolonged immobility. These risk factors include degree of ventricular enlargement (Lonnum and Kornstad, 1974), degree of electroencephalographic abnormality, and degree of psychological (especially language) dysfunction (Kaszniak et al., 1978).

In order to illustrate the personal cost of this common condition, I will describe a recent visit to my great aunts, who are living together since the deaths of their husbands. As we were sitting in their living room in the evening, reminiscing about old times (which they recalled vividly), they suggested we watch television. The women have two TV sets, one beside the other, one belonging to each, and they argued about which gets better reception. We then looked up the evening program fare in the newspaper (rather newspapers—each sister has a subscription to a different local paper). After arguing about which paper had more accurate news, we finally decided to forego television. We reminisced a bit more, but a pause in the conversation led one of my aunts to suggest watching television. An argument again ensued about whose set was better. Against my exhortations, they both retrieved their newspapers and reviewed the available programs. They even made some of the exact same verbal exchanges as previously, "Have you ever seen this show?" "No, I never have, there will never be another program like *Gunsmoke*." "Is *Gunsmoke* on tonight?" "No, I said. . . ." I finally got the newspapers back on top of the respective sets and everybody back in their chairs, but, before five minutes had gone by, one of the women had said, "I wonder what's on TV tonight" and the other had leaped up to check the schedule. "Don't look in the Decatur *Herald*, dear, their TV section is not nearly as good as. . . ."

The first two or three repetitions were humorous, but then a sadness overcame me. These fine old ladies could remember old times perfectly well, but for recent events they were totally oblivious. I imagine for them life is something like walking through darkness with a searchlight illuminating only their immediate location; all the rest is dense blackness, except the far distance behind them which they can see but to where they can never return.

My great aunts, both in their eighties, are both probably suffering from senile dementia of the Alzheimer type. In their cases, like in those of other patients, the knowledge of whether or not they have neurofibrillary tangles in cortical neurons is not worth the expense, trauma, and danger of a brain biopsy. We have ruled out treatable causes. They were taking many medicines, including digitalis, which could have been contributing to the mental decline. "If I can't remember if I've taken my medicine, Lyle," one aunt told me (calling me by my father's name), "I just take two more pills to be sure." Relatives administered the medication for some months, but finally nursing home placement became necessary.

Other Identifiable Causes

The typical stroke patient has devastating motor and sensory symptoms related to a large infarction in the distribution of a specific vessel. These large infarctions may produce significant symptoms and signs of organic mental dysfunction, but do not lead to progressive intellectual deterioration. Some individuals, usually those with severe arterial hypertension, develop many small strokes which lead to dementia. Small episodes of worsening impact characterize the clinical picture; some authors have compared the course of this disorder to walking down a flight of stairs, contrasted to the escalator-smooth descent of other dementias. Probably the best term for this entity is multi-infarct dementia (Hachinski et al., 1974). When the small infarctions are restricted to the deep frontal lobes, the term Binswanger's disease or subcortical arteriosclerotic dementia is sometimes used (Caplan and Schoene, 1978). Actually, vascular experts feel that the pathological changes in the smaller blood vessels represent a vasculopathy that is distinct from arteriosclerosis. A family with this type of vasculopathy not associated with hypertension has been reported (Sourander and Walinder, 1977). Winston Churchill suffered multi-infarct dementia during his second term as Prime Minister, as described in anguishing detail by his family physician, Lord Moran (1966).

Malignant brain tumors, both primary and metastatic, can evidence progressive intellectual deterioration, usually in association with the so-called frontal lobe signs. Although transient improvement follows steroid therapy and future oncological research predicts significant therapeutic breakthroughs, the present prognosis is so dismal that these must be classified as identifiable, but not treatable causes of dementia. In some demented patients, neoplastic cells are so widespread throughout the brain that the pathological diagnosis of gliomatosis cerebri can be made (Sarhaddi et al., 1973). Systemic cancer can sometimes produce dementia without direct spread to the brain. This can occur with multi-focal leukoencephalopathy (Martin and Banker, 1969), or with less defined histopathologic deterioration.

Other systemic disorders present with progressive intellectual deterioration. A very rare patient with Whipple's disease has the pathological process largely restricted to the brain (Romanul et al., 1977). Although antibiotic treatment can counter some of the systemic manifestations of Whipple's disease, no cases with neurological improvement have been reported. In some dialysis centers, a rare patient undergoing chronic hemodialysis develops mental changes, myoclonus, and a characteristic stuttering and hesitation of speech. This entity has been called "dialysis dementia," but its rapid progression and associated findings lead most neurologists to use the less specific eponymic appellation, Alfrey's encephalopathy. Some evidence suggests the symptoms are due to aluminum accumulation in brain tissue (Arieff et al., 1979). Probably the only real treatment is renal transplantation, although diazepam produces transient improvement.

Head trauma is another significant identifiable cause of dementia. Severe dementia with neurological signs can result from a single episode of severe trauma; the mental defect is not progressive. Multiple minor blows can produce a cumulative effect—a very chronic, slowly progressive intellectual and personal deterioration which has been studied extensively in boxers (Corsellis et al., 1973). The stereotype of the punch drunk boxer ("Was that the bell? What round is this?") has a basis in reality. This chronic destruction of a human personality, observed by cheering fans, has received the appellation "dementia pugilistica."

Chronic alcoholism is associated with many different dementing conditions. Pellagra is extremely rare, probably because niacin is naturally present in beer. Korsakov's disease is more common, but its restricted memory loss leads to its classification as an amnestic condition, as already discussed. Subdural hematoma is common among alcoholics. After all these conditions are removed, however, another alcoholic dementia may remain. While unequivocal evidence of this separate entity eludes us, clinical impression describes a mild but global dementia associated with moderate cortical atrophy (Fox et al., 1976). Mental function seems to improve after weeks to months of sobriety. Follow-up CT scans seem to show a reversal of the cortical atrophy (Carlen et al., 1978). Apparent reversal of cortical atrophy has been seen in metabolic conditions which are characterized by shifts within fluid compartments (Heinz et al., 1977).

Jakob-Creutzfeldt disease is a rapidly progressive dementing illness with widespread neurological dysfunction, including ataxia, myoclonus, and cortical degeneration that is so severe that it can occasionally produce cortical blindness. The disorder has been transmitted to chimpanzees and other experimental animals and, unwittingly via corneal transplantation and electrode implantation, to man. The nature of the transmissible agent remains a mystery. A few hypochondriac physicians have refused to accept demented persons as patients because of an hysterical fear of spread of this agent. Neurosurgical procedures and neuropathological examination of Jakob-Creutzfeldt patients require special precautions, but ordinary person-to-person contact should engender no anxiety (Gajdusek et al., 1977).

Huntington's disease is a dominantly inherited disorder that is characterized by dementia and abnormal movements. The underlying pathology involves degeneration of the caudate nucleus, enlarging frontal horns of the lateral ventricles, and allowing suggestive diagnosis by ventricular shape visualized by pneumoencephalography or CT scan (Barr et al., 1978). Dopamine blocking agents, especially haloperidol, improve the abnormal movements but not the mental deterioration. Gamma-aminobutyric acid (GABA) is decreased in brain and CSF of Huntington's disease patients (Manyam et al., 1978). Therapeutic attempts to increase GABA synthesis or decrease its degradation have been largely unsuccessful (Barr et al., 1978), although a few exceptions give hope for future rational therapy (Perry et al., 1979).

A large number of other degenerative brain conditions are characterized by progressive dementia. In general, these disorders are named by eponym, and unequivocal diagnosis requires histological examination of brain tissue. Pick's disease has symptomatology and course similar to Alzheimer's. Neurofibrillary tangles are present in both diseases, but in Pick's disease, atrophy is restricted to anterior frontal and inferior temporal cortices. Clinical differentiation can be attempted based upon the more severe memory loss, and some elements of aphasia (such as word searching and spatial disorientation) in Alzheimer's. The distribution of cortical atrophy visible on CT scan can suggest Pick's disease (McGeachie et al., 1979).

Other degenerative diseases with diagnosis based on histopathology include progressive subcortical gliosis (Neumann and Cohn, 1967), amyloid angiopathy with demyelinative plaques (Heffner et al., 1976), anterior horn cell degeneration with Bunina bodies (Hart et al., 1977), and dementia with intraneuronal Lafora inclusions (Suzuki et al., 1971). Some rare dementias are based upon associated systemic findings, such as the dementia with myopathy reported by Torvik and his co-workers (1974), or the dementia and bony cysts described by Hakula and Iivanainen (1973). Familial dementia with nonspecific histopathologic findings is not uncommon (Schaumburg and Suzuki, 1968), especially among in-bred populations (Cross and McKusick, 1967). Several disorders which mainly occur in childhood can rarely present as progressive dementia in adults. These include gangliosidosis (O'Neill et al., 1978), neuroaxonal dystrophy (Torack and Hughes, 1972), metachromatic leukodystrophy (Bosch and Hart, 1978), and the Cornelia de Lange syndrome (Cherington et al., 1969). Other degenerative diseases which include progressive intellectual decline as a major part of more widespread neurological deterioration include the progressive myoclonic epilepsies, cerebral hemosiderosis (Tomlinson and Walton, 1964), progressive supranuclear palsy (Albert et al., 1974), and some cases of spinocerebellar degeneration.

Although these disorders show clinical differences, the clinician need not make extensive efforts to specify the exact appropriate eponym. Once treatable etiologies have been ruled out, a final diagnosis like "dementia associated with cortical atrophy" seems to be warranted. Arguments about whether a severely deteriorated patient suffers from Alzheimer's or Pick's disease symbolize what is wrong with clinical neurology.

EVALUATION

The recommended evaluation of a demented individual is offered in Table 3. History and examination are included, even though their importance goes without saying. It is a bit demeaning to say, "Don't forget to take a history," but it is so vital to a successful evaluation that repetition is warranted. In our series of demented patients, all five who reverted to normal with discontinuance of drug therapy had the use of drugs uncovered during the history. The laboratory tests should be guided by the history and examination findings. For example, if the patient's gait is completely normal, CT scan could be deleted if the clinician can evaluate resectable mass lesions by other means, such as radionuclide brain scan. On the other hand, if the patient has the wide based, hesitant gait characteristic of NPH, some evaluation of ventricular enlargement and cortical atrophy is essential. If CT scanning is not available, pneumoencephalography should be performed if the patient's general health permits and if uncovered NPH would make him a surgical candidate. Many clinicians feel that a spinal tap in this situation is probably unnecessary (Wells, 1977). The India ink and cryptococcal antigen evaluations are the main reasons for CSF exam, but cryptococcal meningitis always presents with headache and other general symptoms—never with dementia alone. If the various serum tests for syphilis, especially the FTA, are positive, a LP can then be performed for the evaluation of neurosyphilis.

What kind of results can one expect from this rather expensive evaluation? You may recall one or two patients who presented with dementia, but evaluation revealed hypothyroidism or subdural hematoma. This startling victory appears against a background of constant defeat, a faceless, nameless jumble of the demented becoming more so, exasperated families, patients rummaging through drawers in the middle of the night, wandering on the

TABLE 3: Protocol for the Workup of a Patient with Dementia

History:	From relatives as well as the patient, with special attention to alcohol and drug use.
Examination:	Physical, neurological, and mental status.
Blood tests:	CBC, urinalysis, B_{12}, folate, barbiturate and bromide levels, VDRL and FTA, renal, hepatic, and thyroid function tests, electrolytes including calcium.
Laboratory examinations:	Skull x-ray, EEG, radioisotope brain scan, and either CT scan or (general health permitting) pneumoencephalogram. CSF examination with India ink and CSF analysis for cells, protein, glucose, and VDRL.

interstate median, urinating on the sofa, dull eyes, drooling, wives crying, husbands guilty when institutionalization becomes necessary—a gray mass of defeat.

Several published series show that a large minority of patients presenting with progressive intellectual deterioration have an underlying cause that is potentially amenable to therapy. At a general hospital, like Middlesex Hospital in London (Harrison and Marsden, 1977) or the Nashville Veterans Hospital (Freemon, 1976), up to one in three patients has such a cause for his dementia. Tertiary-care speciality centers with a wider referral pattern have a lower ratio, perhaps one in eight (Smith et al., 1976). The most common diagnostic entities causing treatable dementia in four published series are normal pressure hydrocephalus, depression, chronic drug intoxication, and resectable subdural hematoma or meningioma (Figure 2). Your own experience seems to contradict formal reviews because the successfully treated case is not seen again, while the progressively dementing patient returns many times, each time with new or worsening symptomatology.

Unfortunately, not all patients with a potentially amenable etiology respond to therapy. This is especially true with normal pressure hydrocephalus, where only about half of the patients with the clinical and radiologic picture of NPH improve significantly following shunting. Nevertheless, a significant proportion of demented patients have an underlying disorder that should receive specific therapy. Geschwind (1975) has summarized this need in a most forceful manner: "The potentially curable causes of progressive intellectual deterioration represent the most overlooked treatable medical conditions in America."

Since the government pays for much medical care, government leaders

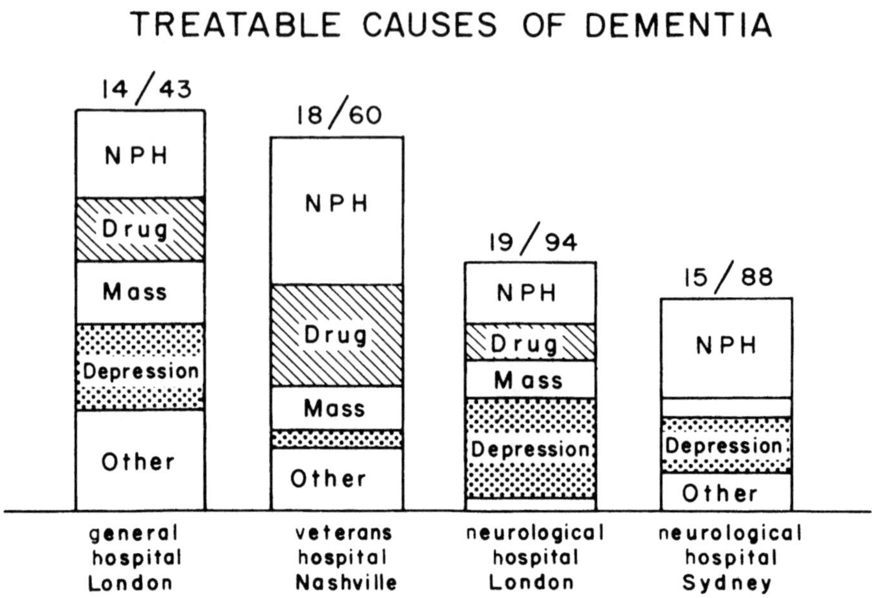

Figure 2: Four consecutive patient series from three countries show that a significant minority of patients with progressive intellectual deterioration have an underlying disease that is potentially amenable to specific treatment. The height of the bar represents the percentage of treatable patients; the fraction is the number of treatable cases over the total number.

often look upon clinical conditions in economic terms. The head of the National Institute of Aging has concluded that a dementia work-up is a valuable expenditure of government funds: "A $500 bill for a diagnostic work-up, including $240 for a CAT scan, is minimal when contrasted with the $15,000 per year one Medicaid nursing home bed costs" (Butler, 1979). Apparently, he has found a location where he can obtain a CT scan at a bargain price.

TREATMENT

The syndrome of dementia exemplifies the ancient principle of medicine—to heal sometimes but to comfort always. A small percentage, probably about a fifth, of demented patients suffer from an underlying medical or neurological illness and show at least a partial response to specific treatment. The nonspecific or comforting treatment that includes counseling to the patient and his family, providing the best possible environment for the patient and treating complications must not be downgraded (Snyder and Harris, 1976).

Counseling given to the patient should probably be more optimistic than that given to the family. Certainly, the patient needs his spouse or another trusted family member to take over his financial affairs. However, the family should try to avoid placing the patient in the "sick role," sitting in a wheelchair while all his needs are met. Rather, he should be encouraged to continue to be as useful and busy as his mental capacity allows. If the dementia results from an hereditary disease such as Huntington's chorea, genetic counseling should be given; many people find the concept of genetic disease with onset in middle to late life difficult to grasp (Shoulson and Fahn, 1979).

Most demented patients do best in the environment that is most familiar to them. Just as their memories for people and events from years gone by are better than those for more recent things, so also the strongest recollections are for objects and rooms with which the patient became familiar many years ago. If the patient has lived at one residence for many years, he will probably do best remaining there. Some patients deteriorate to such a degree that admission to a professional nursing facility becomes absolutely necessary. One can usually predict, however, that further deterioration will follow as the patient copes with a new environment. An exception to the rule of nursing home deterioration is the demented housewife who cannot give up the exhausting demands of running a home to her relatives, but improves in the more regulated environment of the nursing facility.

Of course, the physician treats complications as they arise. Depression, in particular, is frequent. Some people become particularly disoriented at night; night lights and familiar environmental cues help more than sleeping pills. Many clinicians feel that the brain of the demented patient is particularly sensitive to the mildest metabolic derangement, and that the dementia worsens with urinary or respiratory infections and improves following their eradication.

This chapter concludes with a word—a discouraging word—about pharmacological therapy for the dementia syndrome. Well-designed studies have shown that certain pharmacological agents are superior to placebos, but this effect on dementia is slight. Based upon the theory (now discredited) that senile dementia was due to cerebral arteriosclerosis, vasoactive agents were attempted as therapy. Although some studies show cognitive improvement compared to placebo following administration of papaverine (Stern, 1970), cyclanedate (Rao et al., 1977; Capote and Parikh, 1978), or even antiocoagulants (Ratner et al., 1972), an exhaustive review of the research suggests that this slight improvement is due to direct effects of these agents on brain metabolism (Yesavage et al., 1979). A group of ergot derivatives (dihydroergocornine, dihydroergokristine, and dihydroergokryptine) were marketed together because of supposed vasoactive properties; while subsequent investigation has found that this ergot combination has no effect on blood vessels, carefully controlled clinical studies have shown a slight, but definite therapeutic effect on cognitive function in senile dementia (Gaitz et al., 1977).

A wide variety of agents that affect neurotransmitter function can improve intellectual abilities in senile dementia of various etiologies. Well-controlled studies show a slight, but definite clinical improvement following treatment with choline containing phospholipids (Savoldi et al., 1978), with the GABA congener piracetam (Abuzzahab et al., 1977), and with dopaminergic agents such as levodopa (Lewis et al., 1978) and amantadine (Chierichetti et al., 1977). Negative reports, however, have also appeared. It is feared that these new agents will fail the test of clinical experience as have earlier promising therapeutic modalities, such as methylphenidate (Crook et al., 1977), RNA (Munch-Peterson et al., 1974), and hyperbaric oxygenation (Goldfarb et al., 1972). Pharmacological therapy of the dementia syndrome is not a major therapeutic modality—not a major weapon in our therapeutic armamentarium. At best, it is an aid to other supportive measures.

Chapter 9

Aphasia

INTRODUCTION

Aphasia is an acquired disorder of symbolic communication. The victim of aphasia has difficulty producing and understanding speech, reading, and writing. A deaf person who becomes aphasic can no longer produce or understand sign language. The most severely affected patients even have difficulty communicating with gestures (Goodglass and Kaplan, 1963).

The diagnosis of aphasia implies dysfunction of the dominant hemisphere. This is not to say that a wide variety of neurological disorders cannot also affect speech. Both cerebellar and right-hemisphere dysfunction can produce a deficit of prosody, the song-like quality that gives speech its emotional component. Patients with a wide variety of lesions, from cortex to basal ganglia to brain stem, have various pronunciation problems, but this dysarthria is not aphasia. A wide variety of conditions, from catatonia to the locked-in syndrome, produce mutism, but the term aphasia, despite its derivation, is a specific disorder of higher cerebral function and is not applicable to everyone who does not speak.

Some semantic purists dislike the term aphasia, pointing out that some aphasic patients actually produce more speech than normal people do. Others recommend the term dysphasia, but in everyday use this term is frequently mistaken for dysphagia, which means difficulty swallowing. The term aphasia will be used to identify the communication difficulty described in this chapter.

EXAMINATION

One can divide the examination of the aphasia patient into six parts:

1. spontaneous speech,

2. understanding of spoken speech,
3. reading,
4. writing,
5. naming,
6. repetition.

In general, one attempts to gauge the patient's level of function in each of these six areas so that subsequent examination can determine improvement or worsening.

It is essential to evaluate a significant amount of spontaneous speech. For most, but not all, patients, the rendition of the clinical history is sufficient. The physician interested in organic mental disease must listen not only to the message given in the history, but to the way it is delivered as well. The aphasic patient may use abnormal words or engage in circumlocutions around missing words. We all experience word searching (the pause in normal conversation when the mind fails to come up with the next word in sequence), but mildly aphasic individuals can suffer this symptom to an excruciating degree. Great patience is required of the examiner in order to observe while the aphasic talks around an obvious word. If the spouse gives the history with the patient silent, the examiner must bring out the patient on some subject. I obtain best results by asking the patient how the symptomatology related by the spouse affects him. If his halting answers are interrupted by the spouse, the question can be repeated later during the physical examination with the spouse absent. Often an examination finding such as a scar provides a focus of conversation to test spontaneous speech more fully.

If the patient is apparently without speech, perhaps he can say his name or repeat a familiar phrase such as "red, white, and blue." The examiner can try to have the patient join him in a well-known series such as the alphabet or the days of the week. If all else fails, he may be able to relate a syllable, even "yeah" or "nuh," to a shaking of the head. Many aphasiologists have reported that speechless people can hum a tune or even sing the words to a song, especially if they are accompanied by other singers (Yamadori et al., 1977). I have rarely obtained success in this endeavor, even by having the entire ward masquerade as a choir, unless one considers success to be the careful development of a reputation for eccentricity.

Similarly, one defines the patient's ability to understand spoken speech. Perhaps he can follow a simple command like "raise your hand" but not a more complex one like "touch your forehead with your left thumb." Perhaps he can follow one command but not two, or two but not three. The aphasic patient may follow a previous command, not the present one, an abnormal phenomenon subsumed under the general term perseveration (Allison and Hurwitz, 1967).

The examiner also estimates the patient's abilities to read and write. While aphasiologists generally have a special series of written sentences that they use to evaluate reading, the physician who encounters aphasic patients infrequently may utilize a nearby magazine. An approximation of reading ability can be gauged by asking the patient to interpret a newspaper headline. Sports headlines are best avoided, since frequently they are intelligible only to the most avid fan. If the patient cannot read the full headline, perhaps he can read single words or single letters. If he can do none of these, the examiner must be sure the problem is not one of visual acuity. Many severely affected aphasics can write their names. More difficult is writing from dictation and most difficult is composing a spontaneous sentence. A good test for a hospital in-patient is to ask him to write a sentence with the word hospital in it. If the patient produces a written response, check it for errors; aphasic patients often write abnormal or extra letters (Rosati and de Bastiani, 1979).

A test of naming is particularly valuable in the differential diagnosis between normality and mild aphasic language disturbance. Practically all aphasic patients have some difficulty naming, especially parts of things. I usually go through these objects and their parts: finger/nail, wristwatch/face (crystal), belt/buckle, nose/nostril. If the examiner is embarrassed to ask a normal person such seemingly inane questions, he can approach the topic under the guise of memory testing. "Do you have any trouble remembering the names of things? Let's test it. What is this called?"

Most modern aphasiologists contend that the examination of an aphasic person is not complete without a specific evaluation of the patient's ability to repeat. The reasoning behind this supposed requirement lies in an attempt to evaluate the rare but theoretically important disorder of conduction aphasia.

DIAGNOSIS

The diagnostic process for the patient suspected of aphasia is separated into two phases. First, the clinician makes the diagnosis of the aphasia syndrome; he separates those who are truly aphasic from those with other syndromes masquerading as aphasia. Secondly, he determines the cause of the aphasia. What about determining the type of aphasia? With a few caveats described later, little value results from the great effort involved in determining the type of aphasia, since one investigator's classification, distilled from a lifetime of experience, serves another investigator only as a repository of disparaging accusations.

The second diagnostic process will be discussed first, since it is more automatically dealt with. Aphasia indicates ongoing dysfunction of the dominant hemisphere. Usually, other associated signs such as hemiparesis or hemianopsia corroborate hemispheral involvement by the destructive process. One evaluates the patient with aphasia as one would any other patient with focal brain disease. The rate of progression of dysfunction, its severity, and associated symptoms and conditions serve as diagnostic indicators. Roentgenologic and other laboratory tests aid in localization and diagnosis. Destructive lesions produce most instances of aphasia, but aphasic difficulty can rarely be associated with seizure discharge involving the dominant hemisphere (Gascon et al., 1973). All clinicians are familiar with Todd's paralysis—transient hemisparesis following a focal seizure—but many are unaware that transient aphasia can also occur in the same manner; actually Todd's original patient had an association of aphasia and right hemiparesis following epileptic jerking of the right arm and leg.

A more difficult question is, when is a patient aphasic? One must dissociate aphasia from dysarthria, from mutism, from confusion, from delirium. Perhaps the most frequent differentiation is mild aphasia versus normality. A patient has a right hemiparesis and one wonders if his lesion involves speech areas of the left hemisphere. A patient complains of memory loss and one wants to know if this is the specific loss for words. A depressed patient produces very little speech and one hopes to determine if he speaks little because he is depressed or if he is depressed because he cannot speak. These patients with near normal speech need a full language examination as already described. Special attention should be paid to naming (especially naming parts of things) and to immediate verbal memory as evaluated by forward digit span.

A patient with severe pronunciation difficulties can present a diagnostic problem. If this symptom occurs in isolation, the dysarthric can easily be differentiated from the aphasic by handing the patient pad and pencil. Aphasic disorder of speech is, with a few exceptions (such as Dr. Samuel Johnson), associated with characteristic abnormalities of reading and writing. This differential diagnosis usually arises, however, in a patient with a left-hemisphere lesion producing right facial weakness with associated cortical dysarthria and right hemiplegia. The patient without aphasia may need special urging to attempt writing with his left hand; although awkward, he should write easily intelligible full sentences. Cortical dysarthria frequently occurs with aphasia; this patient may produce abnormal and repeated letters and words or simply a series of unintelligible lines and dots. The patient with dysarthria alone will be able to follow commands, even complex ones; but the patient with associated aphasia will have difficulty, especially with commands involving multiple steps or unfamiliar terms.

Some clinicians may have difficulty differentiating the patient who has aphasia that is so severe that he has almost no words from the unresponsive but apparently awake individual. The latter group encompasses akinetic mutism, catatonia, and severe depression. The wordless aphasic patient looks as if he wants to talk. When one addresses him he establishes eye contact spontaneously. Unfortunately, many patients with severe aphasia are also depressed, perhaps reactively at the loss of communicative ability, therefore the diagnosis may not be a simple either/or decision.

Patients who have many words but meaningless rambling speech may be aphasic or they may be confused or demented. Listening carefully to the spontaneous speech will probably differentiate these conditions. The aphasic may have additional or unusual words that at first hearing seem like English words but are not. When asked standard dementia questions, aphasic patients either will not understand at all, will give the correct answer, or will search for the correct term with other words. "The President? He's the guy in Washington who does the leadership, lives in the White House." The confused or demented patient will answer incorrectly or will attempt to hide his lack of knowledge, as we all do when we cannot perform something we think we should.

Severe schizophrenia—so-called "schizophrenic word salad"—has some aspects of aphasia. The clang association—using a rhyming word—is supposedly classic for schizophrenia, but can also be seen in aphasia. Usually associated symptoms make schizophrenia obvious, just as other focal neurological signs, such as a right field cut, make the aphasia easy to recognize. The administration of phenothiazines or haloperidol to a patient who is otherwise impossible to diagnose will almost invariably improve the schizophrenia and may transiently worsen the aphasia.

The most outrageous misdiagnosis I ever encountered concerned a recently divorced woman admitted to a psychiatric hospital because of a conversion reaction. When I saw her in consultation, however, it was obvious that her right hemiplegia was not due to conversion. Although the psychiatrist had attributed her speechlessness to a "resistance to psychotherapy" she was actually severely aphasic. She was depressed, as the psychiatrist had noted, but her depression lifted markedly when the aphasia syndrome was diagnosed and speech therapy begun.

CLASSIFICATION

Imagine how exciting it must have been in the last quarter of the nineteenth century to describe various aphasia syndromes. Ever since the philosophical anatomy of Gall and Spurzheim, medical scientists had attempted to correlate specific mental functions with specific brain regions. Those aspects of behavior that man shares with animals had been disrupted by disease in man and experimental manipulations in animals. A growing understanding of brain lesions which produce paralysis or visual loss contrasted with the speculative nonsense which purported to describe the neurological basis of love, pride, and other higher functions. Medicine had uncovered a specific human capacity, language, with a neurological basis in the brain. It was no wonder that attempts at holistic explanation went beyond the available data. What is surprising, however, is our inability to break away from these early tentative concepts.

Wernicke and subsequent aphasiologists hypothesized that an area of cerebral cortex existed which was responsible for translating sounds into words. This area was thought to be near the cortical auditory analyzer, the termination of medial geniculate fibers in Heschl's gyrus, along the superior margin of the temporal lobe (Figure 1). This region, eponymically honoring Wernicke, has slowly shifted over the years, posteriorly and superiorly (Bogen and Bogen, 1976). Sound waves transduce changes in neural firing rates by the organ of Corti. These normal impulses are transmitted via the cochlear nerve and nucleus, lateral lemniscus, medial geniculate body, and thalamocortical radiations, to Heschl's gyrus as described in Chapter 2. Neural events within the cortical neurons of Wernicke's area correspond to the recognition by the mind of the original spoken word. Perhaps, say some aphasiologists, certain portions of Wernicke's area are responsible for certain types of words. For example, the most posterior extent may be the neural representation for the names of body parts and the names of colors. The superior parietal lobule, said Gerstmann (carrying this idea almost to its extreme), contains the names of the five fingers.

Early aphasiologists contrasted this posterior speech region with the third frontal gyrus already identified as important for language by Broca. This region, it was thought, controlled motor behavior by sending fibers via basal ganglia and reticular substance to the anterior horn cells and analogous primary motor neurons of cranial nerves. Today we speak of motor engrams triggered by the activity in Broca's region; engrams which interact with motor-related portions of the brain to affect the contraction and relaxation of speech-related musculature to produce a series of sounds that are meaningful as words and sentences to the speaker and to others.

According to this basic theory, lesions of this hypothetical posterior region will produce difficulty understanding because of a disruption of the neural representation of auditory word memories. The victim of this lesion will be unable to name objects he sees because of a disruption of the associated visual word memories. He will be unable to repeat things because he will not understand or register what he hears. His spontaneous speech will be quite fluent (even near normal), except that he may pause to search for words which are not readily retrieved from the disrupted word memories. Lesions of the hypothetical anterior region, on the other hand will produce a subject who can understand everything but can produce few, if any, words. A large lesion involving both these regions produces a global language deficit.

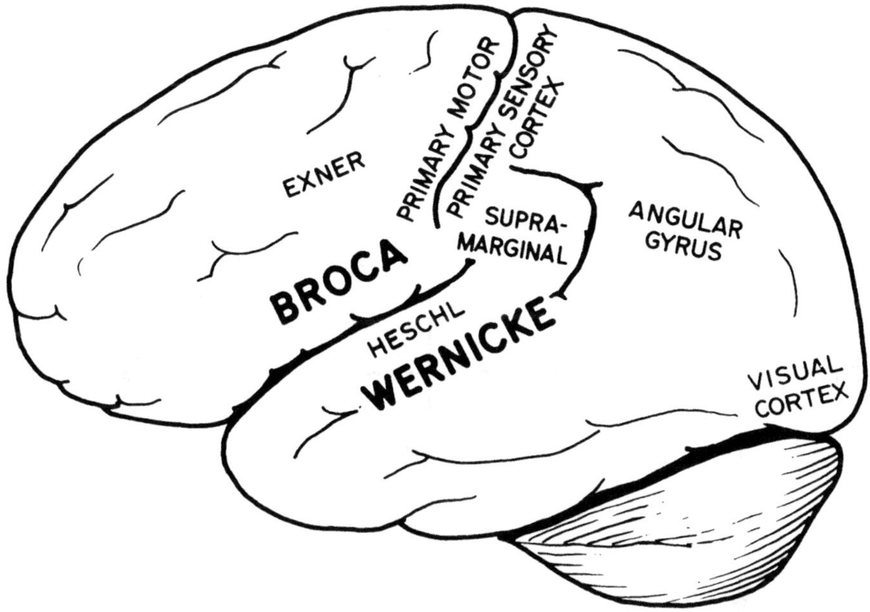

Figure 1: The eponymic cortical regions related to language have ill-defined borders and in the case of Wernicke's area even an ill-defined center.

It was natural for neuroanatomists to connect these theoretical regions with pathways and to imagine the results of disconnection. The accompanying diagram (Figure 2) from Lichtheim's famous paper of 1885 is an example. He draws the "centre of auditory images" and the "centre of motor images" connected by a reflex arc. If this connection is broken, the subject could understand but not repeat—so-called conduction aphasia. If one isolates both speech regions from the rest of the brain, or in Lichtheim's terms, the place where concepts are elaborated, one produces isolation aphasia where the patient can repeat but has little real knowledge of what he is saying. Later in his article, Lichtheim added reading and writing to his schema, producing a diagram too complex for modern generations. Reading implied a posterior center for visual word symbols; writing an anterior region called Exner's area which controlled hand and arm muscles to produce written communication symbols analogous to the control over speech musculature exerted by Broca's area.

The concept of basic types of aphasia which can be differentiated along the anterior-posterior axis of the left hemisphere seems to appear in almost all neurological writings (but not in linguistic formulations which argue from a grammar base, without reference to the brain). Some use the terms motor and sensory aphasia or even their modern synonyms—output and

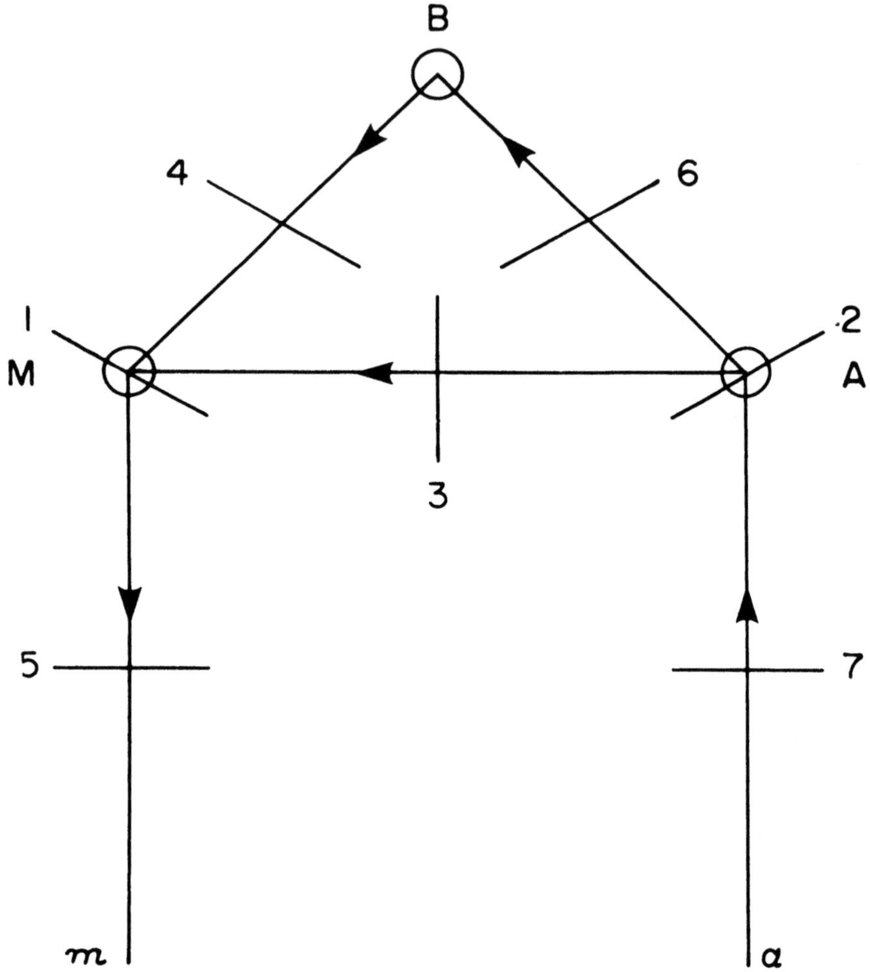

Figure 2: "We may call centre of auditory images and centre of motor images, respectively, the parts of the brain where these memories are fixed," explained Lichtheim (1885) referring to the neural representation of words. "They are designated in this schema by the letters A and M. The reflex arc consists of an afferent branch aA which transmits the acoustic impressions to A; and an efferent branch Mm, which conducts the impulses from M to the organs of speech; and is completed by the commissure binding together A and M. When intelligence of the imitated sounds is superimposed, a connection is established between the auditory centre A, and the part where concepts are elaborated, B. The next step in the formation of volitional or intelligent speech involves a centrifugal connection between B and M." Lichtheim (1885) went on to even more fanciful diagrams and explanations.

input. Others use the terms expressive and receptive, but these are not ideal since the posterior aphasic may show such hesitation and word searching that his deficit could be described as expressive. Schuell and her co-workers (1964) devised five types of aphasia, based upon response to speech therapy. Types 1, 4, and 5 correspond to mild, moderate, and severe global or total aphasia. Group 3 corresponds to the more anterior lesion, and Group 2 to the more posterior. Geschwind (1971) introduced the term nonfluent to signify the anterior aphasic with few words, and the term fluent for a series of aphasic syndromes most of which are associated with posterior lesions. Published studies which classify aphasics into groups based upon clinical examination, determine lesion site by radioisotope imaging (brain scan) or by computed tomography (CT scan), and attempt a correlation, generally corroborate a significant clinical difference between anterior and posterior lesions (Karis and Horenstein, 1976; Naeser and Hayward, 1978). Table 1 summarizes this dichotomy.

ANTERIOR APHASIA

The patient with destruction of the left frontal lobe has a paucity of spontaneous speech. He may be almost completely mute or may communicate with very few words. His understanding, while not normal, is relatively preserved. Almost all patients with an anterior aphasia have an associated right hemiplegia as well as an associated right face and tongue weakness, which causes those words which are produced to be slurred. This slurring, referred to as cortical dysarthria, can be so severe that the examiner has great difficulty interpreting the patient's speech attempts. A difficult differential diagnosis, already discussed, attempts to determine if the cortically dysarthric individual is also aphasic or not. Most patients with aphasia due to frontal lesions have difficulty mimicking motor acts, particularly those involving lips and tongue. The frequent association of this oral apraxia with

TABLE 1: Dichotomous Aphasia Classification

Anatomy	Anterior	Posterior
Physiology	Motor	Sensory
Psychology	Expressive	Receptive
Eponym	Broca	Wernicke
Schuell (1964)	Group 3	Group 2
Geschwind (1971)	Nonfluent	Fluent

aphasia has led many to think of anterior aphasia as a verbal apraxia (Trost and Canter, 1974).

Let us examine a specific case, a 29-year-old plumber in perfect health, without significant family history of medical problems or poor medical habits, except for the occasional use of amphetamines for aid in working through the night. While talking to a friend, the patient noted that he was occasionally slurring words. This difficulty progressed over half an hour until he was virtually speechless. At that time, he noted that his right hand was weak. He tried to write *call an ambulance* with his left hand, but only got out a childish scribble, with only the letters CA definitely discernable. While en route to the hospital, his right hand weakness progressed slowly to a complete right hemiplegia. He never lost consciousness.

Examination showed the obvious motor abnormality of right hemiplegia involving the face. The patient could shake his head to indicate yes and no, but could not make any sound. A gutteral exhaled breath was as close as he could come to an attempt to hum a tune. He could follow one command easily and two with some difficulty, but three produced an ironic half smile and a shrug of the shoulders. His attempts at writing with the left hand were restricted to a few straight lines. When given a list of three-letter words like zoo and bee and asked to point at a particular one, he did so unerringly. He could also point at a word that rhymed with a particular choice or could pick a word from a definition or property. "Point at the thing that makes honey." He had an apraxia for tongue and mouth movements and even had some difficulty reproducing complex finger postures of the left hand. He was slightly frightened but alert, cooperative, and not depressed. He laughed when the examiner told a joke and his right facial weakness temporarily disappeared.

The CT scan showed a small hemorrhage, perhaps slightly larger than a golf ball, centering in Broca's area (Figure 3). There was a small ring of edema around the hematoma. Cerebral arteriography showed an early draining vein from the hematoma region, suggesting that a small arteriovenous malformation had produced the hemorrhage.

After approximately one month of speech therapy, the patient was able to clearly say several words and even a few common phrases. Two months after the onset, he could print full sentences with his left hand, although he made frequent errors such as toothbrusk for toothbrush and tattlestore for an undetermined word. Now about six months later, the patient, when calm, speaks almost normally, except his speech has no prosody; each word is spoken separately without emotion. When excited or hurried, however, he begins hesitating and searching for words and can become almost wordless.

Mohr and his co-workers (1978) have reviewed all reported cases of so-called Broca's aphasia and found they fall into two groups:

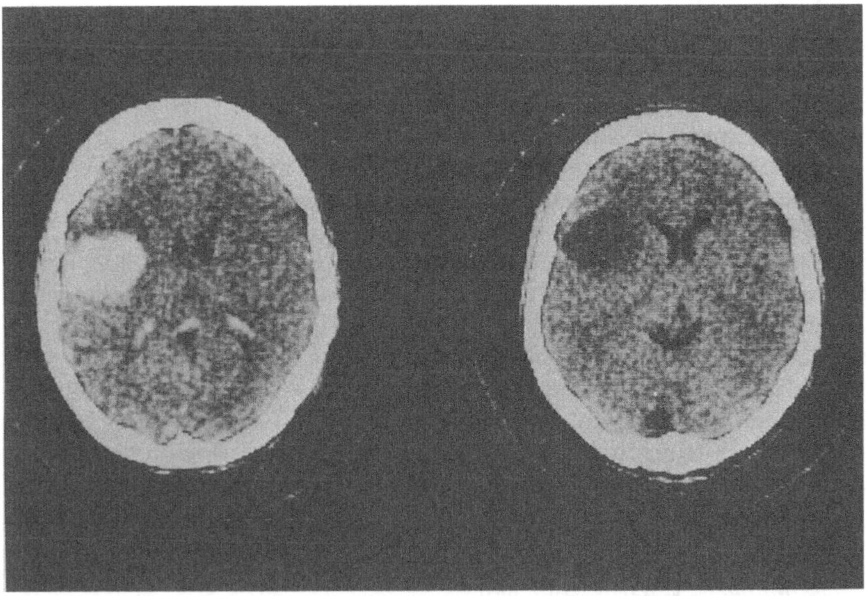

Figure 3: A young man is unable to speak a single word because of an intracerebral hemorrhage (CT scan on left). Four months later the patient's speech production is quite extensive though Broca's area appears to be damaged (right). Neither CT scan is enhanced by intravenous injection of contrast material.

1) patients with large lesions who are initially globally aphasic, improve markedly in understanding, but remain speechless or nearly so; and
2) patients with small frontal lesions who are initially speechless, but recover speech function rather rapidly.

The patient just discussed falls into the second group. Mohr and his colleagues recommend dropping the eponym of Broca, since long-standing nonfluent or Broca's aphasia results from large lesions, while destruction of Broca's area does not produce so-called Broca's aphasia.

POSTERIOR APHASIA

A posterior lesion produces a patient who has considerable amounts but abnormal forms of speech; he uses abnormal or inappropriate words. He may or may not be aware of these errors. He almost always has difficulty naming common objects held before him. He may perseverate in naming, so that the first object is correctly named, but all subsequent ones only invoke the name of the first item. Occasionally, a patient with great word searching will be so aware of his difficulty that he will be reluctant to express himself, thereby masquerading as a patient with a more anterior lesion. Posterior aphasics also have great difficulty following commands. The tendency to ask for repetitions often causes the physician to raise his voice. These patients often are not hemiplegic, but may have an associated hemianopsia.

These cases are sometimes difficult to describe; a recorded interview is a helpful illustration. The patient is a 64-year-old man with the sudden onset one week earlier of a left parietal infarction, confirmed by computed tomography. He had no hemiplegia, but had an incomplete right-field defect on visual-field testing by confrontation. Ophthalmology consultants were unable to confirm this field defect, reporting that their examination was clouded by "poor patient cooperation." Note that in this interview, the patient not only fails to understand the examiner, but he does not even seem to know when the examiner is speaking. Some words made no sense to the transcriber, who wrote the words which sounded most like the patient's production, followed by the word mumbled in parentheses.

Examiner: "What is your name?"

Patient: "Well, uh, I don't know, I guess. They'll be somebody who will come in and get them ready for the service fair (mumbled), I mean, there will be a plate on it. 'Cause I don't know how many people we are going to expect. They will read up and expidate (mumbled) up. There will be a better place. Really."

Examiner: "Listen, I . . ."

Patient: (interrupting) "Yes, sir."

Examiner: "I would like to ask you your age. How old are you?"

Patient: "Well, I don't know, they really gonna be some little pretty bunny billie (mumbled) together to somebody who knows what we can come in, about the Jesus (mumbled) thing."

Examiner: (after a long pause) "Yes?"

Patient: "I mean it will be a little baby" (voice trailing off, last word might have been "maybe").

Examiner: "Let's test your ability to name things."

Patient: (interrupting at end of examiner's sentence) "I appreciate it cause I expect we'll see somebody else" (laughs).

Examiner: "What is this?" (a pencil).

Patient: (taking pencil and holding it in his left hand, taking an envelope lying nearby as if to write on it) "Well, I imagine that's probably, it's you, you play it one way or the other, that's the first time I know it would be."

Examiner: "Good. Now what is this?" (taking away pencil and handing him a closed safety pin).

Patient: "This is just what they regulate (opening pin), what it does mean another plea money (mumbled), suggest I don't know how you would be, so I would, catch say it (mumbled), would be a little free of president (mumbled), what's he gonna, just remember and look at Topeka (mumbled), so you'll just have some unavailable purpose leaping (mumbled). They got to admit that that's the way we will be" (closing pin).

Examiner: "What's this?" (scissors).

Patient: (taking scissors in left hand and opening them) "Well (coughing), I don't know, how you could mail this, places, where could I. (Examiner hands patient a piece of paper and he cuts it with the scissors in several places.) Could I, this here is just, we, we gonna have to see what's going to go."

The patient at this point put down the scissors, spontaneously got up and left the room going back to his own room on the ward.

On other occasions, examination showed that, with concentration, the patient could repeat his name and the phrase "Nashville, Tennessee," but not the phrase "no ifs, ands, or buts." He could not read, nor could he name letters. Asked to write his name, he held the pen in his left hand curled, put pen to paper, but never made more than a dot, despite much urging.

Some have taken the concept of "word-memories" neurally represented in the left parietal lobe one step further, by separating these hypothetical word representations by sensory modalities. The traditional auditory word memories are supposedly located near the termination of the auditory system, as already discussed. Tactile word memories—the ability to name things based upon their feel—are located near the somatosensory termination in the postcentral gyrus. Visual word memories—the ability to name an object observed—are neurally represented at the junction of parietal and occipital lobes. One could then suppose a lesion involving part of the posterior speech region which affected one modality of naming more than another; such patients have been described (Spreen et al., 1966). While if true, this model would have great importance to any attempt to delineate the relation of thinking about objects by the mind to neural activities within the brain, its only immediate practical application involves the methodology by which one tests naming. Frequently, when the examiner holds an object in front of a patient and asks its name, the patient reaches out and touches it. Correct naming after feeling an object represents different neuropsychological capabilities than naming after only seeing the object.

Some call this phenomenon agnosia. A patient who can name an object after feeling it but not by just seeing it (assuming normal visual acuity), suffers visual agnosia. The reverse is tactile or stereoagnosia. Auditory agnosia is a bit more difficult to test; a patient who could not identify a whistle by its sound but who could name it when seeing or touching a referee's whistle has auditory agnosia. Such a patient with normal audiometric testing might be expected to have great difficulty understanding words. Maximum auditory agnosia has been called "pure word deafness"; while most cases are due to bilateral lesions in the cortical terminations of the auditory system, some patients have been described with lesions in that portion of Wernicke's area next to Heschl's gyrus (Newcombe et al., 1978).

OTHER TYPES OF APHASIA

Conduction Aphasia

Conduction aphasia is a syndrome characterized by near-normal understanding of spoken speech and written material, extensive speech production (although this spontaneous speech may be broken by word searching), and a marked difficulty in repeating spoken words. In 1874, Wernicke predicted the existence of such a syndrome by hypothesizing a breaking of the connection between the "understanding area" of the parietal lobe and the speech production engrams in the third frontal convolution. Many aphasiologists have reported that this syndrome is not rare. An excellent review of conduction aphasia by Green and Howes (1977) emphasizes complexities unimagined by Wernicke.

While most accept the idea that conduction aphasia is produced by cutting the arcuate fasciculus between Wernicke's and Broca's areas, Kleist (1962) offers an alternative explanation. Perhaps damage to the left parietal lobe produces, at first, a typical posterior aphasia, but improvement is associated with the development of language capabilities by the right parietal lobe. Understanding has improved greatly, but the pathway from the right parietal lobe to the left frontal lobe is too indirect, or must traverse damaged tissue, so that simple repetition is not possible. Benson and co-workers (1973) suggest that differentiation of these two subsyndromes of conduction aphasia is possible on clinical grounds. Those aphasics with lesions of the arcuate fasciculus cannot mimic motor activities, such as driving a nail or, more particularly, motor acts using lips and tongue. Supposedly, this apraxic deficit results from the severing of the connection between the "idea" of a movement that is isomorphic to neural elements in the parietal lobe, and the motor engrams for the movement in the frontal lobe. The apraxic deficit does not occur with the second type of conduction aphasia, presumably because the "idea" originates in the right parietal lobe and is transmitted directly to the right frontal lobe, then perhaps via the corpus callosum to the left frontal lobe. I imagine that if Lichtheim were alive today he would greatly enjoy diagraming this explanation.

Alexia without Agraphia

Alexia without agraphia is not a rare syndrome. It is overlooked because many patients do not complain of reading difficulty after a stroke; if they do, it is assumed to be a problem of vision. This syndrome usually results from an infarction in the distribution of the left posterior cerebral artery, but can also be produced by a brain tumor in the same region (Cohen et al., 1976). The infarction involves the left occipital lobe, adjacent portions of the left parietal lobe, and the posterior portion of the corpus callosum. Almost all of these patients have a right homonymous hemianopsia and most have a mild naming difficulty. They can generally write fairly well, but are totally unable to read. They cannot read newspaper headlines or even single words, although some can identify single letters. The most startling deficit is their inability to read material that they have themselves written just a few minutes before. They do not even recognize their own signatures.

One explanation for the syndrome involves a disconnection hypothesis (Vincent et al., 1977). The right occipital lobe sees the reading material, but cannot transmit it to the left hemisphere because of the lesion in the posterior part of the corpus callosum. According to this model, no regular pathway exists to carry this information to the right frontal lobe across the intact anterior portion of the corpus callosum. Cases with the full syndrome, but without clear anatomical discontinuity have been reported (Fincham et al., 1975). An alternative theory suggests that the left occipital lobe is responsible for visual exploration of written words (Caplan and Hedley-White, 1974) and its destruction involves failure to appreciate the proper relation of adjacent items, such as letters (Levine and Calvano, 1978).

Gerstmann's Syndrome

Supposedly, destruction of the left posterior parietal lobe produces a characteristic tetrad of symptoms: finger agnosia, right-left confusion, dysgraphia, and dyscalculia (Gerstmann, 1940). Unfortunately, these symptoms do not particularly cluster together to form a specific complex, and, therefore, Gerstmann's syndrome as a separate entity is mainly of historical interest. Nevertheless, it remains something for attending physicians to philosophize over and must be included in a book about organic mental syndromes.

Difficulty with the identification of left and right is common with diseases of either hemisphere. It is even reported by about 10 percent of the general populace, occurring more frequently in women (Wolf, 1973). Finger agnosia, the inability to name particular fingers such as index or ring, is part of the general naming difficulty that occurs with dominant hemisphere dysfunction (Poeck and Orgass, 1969). Abnormalities of calculation and difficulties with reading and writing also occur regularly in aphasic persons, but localization to a particular small portion of the parietal lobe is not warranted by existing clinicopathological material (Critchley, 1966).

While the four symptoms of Gerstmann's syndrome do occur with dominant parietal lobe dysfunction, they do not form a special symptom complex unassociated with other aphasic difficulties.

Apraxia

Apraxia is defined as the inability to perform a series of motor movements in the absence of paralysis, weakness, or uncoordination (Denny-Brown, 1958). A classic example given by Schuell and her colleagues (1964) involves the apraxic patient who wanted a bottle of Coca-Cola. He took the bottle in one hand and the opener in the other, but couldn't quite remember the motor actions necessary to remove the bottle cap. This type of symptom is frequently associated with aphasia. In fact, aphasia may itself be an apraxia of speech musculature. Anterior aphasics, in particular, have difficulty with movements of oral and facial muscles (Mateer and Kimura, 1977).

Difficulty reproducing figures—so-called constructional apraxia—is a completely different phenomenon. This disorder of spatial concepts occurs predominantly with right-hemisphere lesions and is discussed in the next chapter. To differentiate constructional apraxia from the phenomenon under discussion, some preface apraxia with the adjectives ideational or ideomotor, meaning difficulty translating the idea of a motor action into that actual movement. The field of aphasia is complicated by a series of terms of varying definition, so to avoid criticism by book reviewers, I had better point out that some authors search for differences between ideational and ideomotor apraxia (see, for example, Heilman, 1973).

In practice, it is difficult to separate apraxia from agnosia. These terms reflect the deep rut of neurological thinking from the Bell-Magendie discovery of the 1820s. Apraxia is a motor-related phenomenon; agnosia is its sensory equivalent. One could say that the patient with the Coca-Cola bottle had an agnosia for a bottle opener. Some aphasiologists, beginning with Pierre Marie, cut this Gordian knot by using one term, apractagnosia.

Miscellaneous Aphasias

There is almost a limitless number of "types" of aphasia. Lichtheim opined that if he could draw a line between two theoretical brain centers, there must be a syndrome corresponding to the cutting of that connection. Cutting all cortical input to Broca's area except the arcuate fasciculus from Wernicke's area, supposedly gives a typical anterior aphasia with the ability to repeat language retained—so-called transcortical motor aphasia. The vast majority of the readers of this book would benefit from immediately suppressing the phrases transcortical motor and transcortical sensory and never again bringing them to conscious awareness.

Isolation of the speech area sounds at first like a totally theoretical nightmare. The patient sits quietly, never speaking. When he is addressed, he merely parrots back exactly what he hears or the last few words of it. He is a total verbal automaton with auditory system, Wernicke's area, arcuate fasciculus, Broca's area, and motor speech engrams intact, but nothing else. Such a syndrome has been reported as part of a dementing or toxic disease, which relatively spares the speech areas. Carefully studied cases have been reported by Geschwind and co-workers (1968) and by Haiganoosh Whitaker (1976). These patients can occasionally name an object but are usually mute until addressed, at which time they merely repeat most or all of the proffered question. They can continue a familiar series begun by the examiner such as counting. When repeating test sentences, they usually follow the same intonation or emphasis used by the examiner. Of greatest interest is the patient's ability to echo the examiner but to correct his grammar:

Examiner: She has four childs.
Patient: She has four children.

Isolation aphasia, although more a part of the dementia syndrome than an aphasia *sensu strictu*, remains a fascinating aspect of pathological language function.

Almost all aphasics have some difficulty naming things. If this symptom occurs in isolation, it is called nominal or amnestic aphasia. While localizationists aver this syndrome occurs only or predominantly with lesions of the angular gyrus of the parietal lobe, electrical stimulation studies suggest that naming difficulty can occur with dysfunction anywhere in the cortical language system (Whitaker and Ojemann, 1977). Some clinicians use the term central aphasia as a synonym for conduction aphasia, while others use the term differently. Pure word deafness has been described under posterior aphasia, as have the various agnosias. I feel the reader's interest beginning to wane so let us bring to a close this largely idiosyncratic area and try to summarize what, if anything, we have covered of importance.

PRACTICAL IMPORTANCE

It is most important to recognize that a patient is aphasic. The existence of aphasia implies dysfunction of the left hemisphere, and this dysfunction may be countered by standard medical and surgical therapies once the etiology is determined. Of less importance is the localizing value of the two major types of aphasia, indicating anterior versus posterior lesions. The recognition that a patient's difficulty lies in language function permits a much greater understanding of his predicament. One can assure the relatives that the patient is not demented and will not need custodial care for mental reasons. While the patient may have difficulty understanding, it is not because he is hard of hearing; his relatives should not shout at the patient, but should rather restate their directives in simpler terms.

The communication abilities of the aphasic patient who is almost wordless will probably not be amplified by attempts at writing, but some severely affected persons can communicate with a picture board which allows the patient to point at the picture of an item he desires. The clinician can treat associated depression without destroying the doctor-patient relationship by assuming that speechlessness is a "resistance to psychotherapy."

Speech therapy aims to build upon the patient's strengths in order to increase his communication abilities. Those patients who do not recognize their own errors in conversation are least likely to benefit from speech therapy. A near-speechless person will usually get a considerable lift of his depressed spirits when the speech therapist teaches him to reproduce a few frequently used phrases such as "see you around" or "fine, how are you?" He may even speak the phrase at inappropriate times. Everyone who has traveled in a foreign country has noted that much of everyday communication can be accomplished with a very limited set of phrases, the key one being, "quantos pesos?" While the pessimistic cynic claims that the speech therapist does little more than the patient's spouse, there is no doubt in my mind that he provides much of value not readily available to many aphasics. It is not unusual to see an aphasic who has made no attempt to communicate for years improve greatly following intensive speech therapy; it is not surprising that his speech abilities have not changed while they remain unused.

Most of what is known about aphasia has been garnered from patients who speak Western languages. Western thought is characterized by chronological step-by-step analysis. Many tribal groups think only in two basic time periods: long, long ago, and right now. Their languages mirror this thought pattern without the myriad of time tenses of Western languages. One might suspect that left hemisphere lesions in these peoples could produce vastly different symptomatology. Studies of the reading of traditional Chinese characters by aphasics have shown a more complex deficit than originally predicted from the study of Western languages (Sasanuma, 1975). Perhaps, a written language with a pictorial basis involves the spatial hemisphere in language function during learning, and, therefore, less speech deficit follows a subsequent left hemisphere lesion (April and Tse, 1977).

The practical value of a doctor understanding the basics of aphasia is certainly apparent. The deeper meaning of normal and abnormal language function continues to elude our search.

FAMOUS APHASICS

Some of the principles presented in this chapter can be reviewed by a brief survey of some famous aphasics. In some cases, we can only note the existence of aphasia, but in others voluminous historical documentation allows more detailed analysis.

Oscar Wilde was speechless during the last few hours of his life, due to a ruptured left temporal lobe abscess acquired from a middle ear infection. While we do not have any details concerning the speech deficit, we can note the double irony of the aphasic death of the greatest conversationalist of his time and the fatal ear disease of the son of a pioneer of otolaryngology (Freemon, 1971).

Samuel Johnson suffered a stroke at the age of 73 which affected his speech greatly but his writing little. Although he made such frequent verbal errors that he was reluctant to speak at all, several letters are extant which show that he wrote rather well even at the height of his illness. Detailed evaluation of these letters by Critchley (1962) shows that post-stroke letters were generally shorter, had fewer words, and fewer semicolons than pre-stroke letters. Review of his original manuscripts shows that Dr. Johnson made typical substitution errors which he corrected himself upon rereading. For example, his sentence that he had "considered that perhaps death was at hand" was originally written with the words "could not" in the place of "considered." Critchley feels that the slight effect of the stroke on Johnson's writing was due to the overlearning of language in this linguistic genius.

The satirist Jonathan Swift, probably Johnson's equal in the use of words, suffered a stroke while he was in his 70s that left him severely aphasic. He continued to communicate with gestures, particularly with a characteristic shrug of the shoulders which had been his habitual symbol for resignation. He retained a few perseverative phrases only. His editor described Swift's aphasia:

> He again endeavored, with a good deal of pain, to find words, but at last, after many efforts, not being able, he fetched a deep sigh . . . He shrugged up his shoulders and said, "I am what I am, I am what I am," and in about six minutes, repeated the same words two or three times (quoted by Riese, 1959).

Charles Baudelaire, the French poet and bohemian of the middle of the nineteenth century, suffered a typical anterior aphasia (Riese, 1977). Baudelaire is famous to the modern generation for his early descriptions of the subjective effects of marihuana. After his stroke, Baudelaire had only one phrase, pronounced "cre nom nom," a rearrangement of "sacre nom de Dios." This paraphasia was apparently considered to be a religious blasphemy in those days; when he was discharged from the hospital, the nursing sisters sprinkled his room with holy water.

The most famous self-description of aphasia is that of Jacques Lordat, a physiologist of Montpellier medical school. After recovery from an unexplained aphasia, Lordat described his symptoms with these words (translated by Riese, 1954):

> When I wanted to speak I could not find the right expression . . . My thoughts were ready, but the sounds that should convey them to my informant were no longer at my disposal . . . I was no longer able to grasp the ideas of others, for the amnesia that prevented me from speaking made me incapable of understanding the sounds I heard quickly enough to grasp their meaning.

The composer Maurice Ravel slowly became aphasic although it seems that his problem was a poorly understood degenerative condition, rather than a clearly defined infarction. Ravel was an unusual composer, more cerebral than emotional, who attempted to bring careful analysis to his musical works. Ravel's most popular production, *Bolero*, was created for reasons of technical perfection, the world's longest crescendo without harmonic or melodic variation. "I have written only one masterpiece, the *Bolero*," said Ravel, "unfortunately, it contains no music." Ravel's language deterioration, described by his physician Alajouanine (1948) as a Wernicke's aphasia, was associated with a loss of musical talent. This contrasts with a more emotional composer, Shebalin, who wrote complete symphonies after a left hemisphere stroke had left him essentially without speech (Luria et al., 1965).

Chapter 10

Dysfunction of the Minor Hemisphere

INTRODUCTION

Physicians seldom appreciate the diagnostic value of right-hemisphere psychological dysfunction. While most internists recognize the value of aphasia in localizing a lesion to the left hemisphere; few utilize analogous lateralized symptoms pointing to involvement of the right hemisphere. Psychiatrists often rely on formal neuropsychological testing, waiting days or even weeks for the final report, when a few minutes of bedside evaluation might give an immediate and direct diagnosis. Even some neurologists and neurosurgeons who will spend thousands of dollars to obtain laboratory confirmation of focal brain disease fail to fully appreciate the localizing value of right-hemisphere psychological dysfunction.

In a neuropsychological context, the right hemisphere is called the minor or nondominant hemisphere. These terms, which seem to have a pejorative connotation, evolve from the importance of the left hemisphere for speech. If we lived in a different type of society, say one where silent hunters tracked animals through complex forests and swamps, we might say that the right hemisphere was the major one, dominant for spatial abilities; the left hemisphere was only of recreational value relating stories of the hunt around the campfire. In the book, however, we will continue to refer to the left hemisphere as major or dominant, while recognizing the inadequacy of these terms to describe complex intercerebral relationships.

Not long after the recognition of the importance of the left hemisphere for speech, perceptive clinicians began to appreciate the special abilities of the right hemisphere (Benton, 1977). In 1876, Hughlings Jackson described a patient with a right parietal tumor who showed visual disorientation, dressing apraxia, and poor facial recognition. Jackson termed this dysfunction "imperception." These ideas were not accepted by the mainstream of neurology, however, despite a series of corroborating case reports. In the early years of the 20th century, Babinski (1914) described denial of hemiplegia, which he called "anosognosia." It is surprising that the striking clinical findings in these patients did not evoke greater interest; how many of these patients over the years were dismissed as "hysterical?" Only now are we beginning to appreciate this psychological dysfunction, and to evaluate and treat it appropriately. As recently as the early 1960s, the basic neuroscience course in my medical school accepted the theory that the right hemisphere was (psychologically speaking) a "spare" for language up to early childhood. After its "spare" function was lost with the solidification of language in the left hemisphere, the right hemisphere controlled the left side of the body, but had no direct or special function for the individual's mental life.

Two patients taught me the value of understanding right hemisphere dysfunction. The first was a stroke patient who recovered rather well from a left hemiplegia. On his first day home from the hospital, he attempted a walk around the block. Despite the fact that he had made this same walk each evening for many years, he got lost and had to ask a neighbor to walk him home. He could have benefited from counseling about potential difficulties at hospital discharge. The second patient underwent surgical removal of a right hemisphere tumor. His family reported that he had a very poor appetite in the immediate postoperative period. When several appetite stimulants failed, the problem was uncovered by means of closer observation. After each meal, the patient's tray showed that he had consumed only the right half of each dish. The remaining half had been interpreted by the family as poor appetite. This was treated by merely rotating the tray whenever the patient thought he was done eating.

RIGHT HEMISPHERE DYSFUNCTION

Spatial Disorientation

The patient with a lesion of the right cerebral hemisphere has difficulty with spatial concepts. He gets lost easily, perhaps even in his own house. The patient cannot copy designs (Figure 1). This inability to construct geometrical figures is called constructional apraxia, although it has little if anything in common with the ideational or ideomotor apraxia discussed in the previous chapter. Some of these patients have special difficulty with objects in the left visual field even if no hemianopsia is present. A classic example is the failure of the chess player with a right hemisphere stroke to guard against

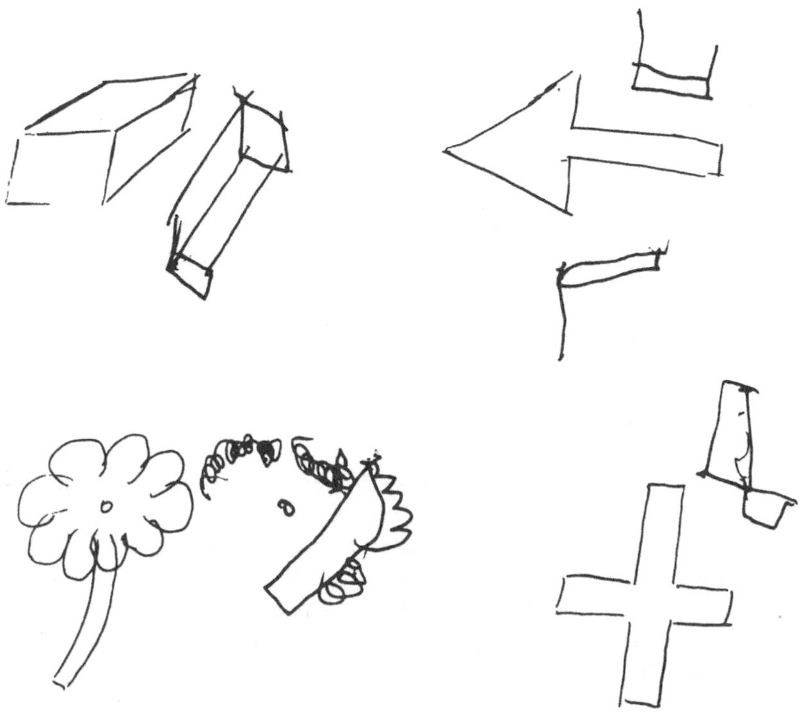

Figure 1: A patient with a right hemisphere lesion has difficulty copying common objects. He has special difficulty with the left side of things, for example the flower or the point of the arrow.

an attack mounted by an opponent on the left side of the chess board (Cherington, 1974).

Indifference to Left Hemiplegia

A few patients with right hemisphere dysfunction claim that the left side of their body is not their own. If they are hemiplegic from the same right hemisphere lesion, they may deny this obvious motor deficit. More commonly, the patient demonstrates a bland indifference to the location, condition, and existence of his left arm. This phenomenon has been graphically demonstrated by the novelist Eric Hodgins, who described his own sudden stroke:

> I commanded myself to get off the floor, and in this I succeeded. I was not dizzy, nothing was spinning, I had no headache or other pain, but my gait was most peculiar; I needed a wall. Something

> kept banging against my left leg. I discovered it to be my left hand and arm, but this was so incomprehensible that a dozen visual reverifications could not explain to me why these were now *things* external to my body (Hodgins, 1963).

Some patients show a disinclination to dress the left side of the body. If they have managed to get the left arm through the sleeve of a blouse (perhaps with help), the shirt buttoning may be irregular, and the patient looks like a young child who has dressed himself for the first time. This has been called dressing apraxia but, like constructional apraxia, has nothing to do with the apraxia associated with aphasia.

Musical Appreciation

At one time, music appreciation was thought to be predominantly or even solely a right hemisphere function (Wertheim, 1969). The composer Shebalin wrote complete symphonies after a left hemisphere stroke left him severely aphasic (Luria et al., 1965). Musical abilities, however, are too complex to be localized to specific brain areas and some aspects, especially sequential analysis, are disrupted by left hemisphere lesions (Gates and Bradshaw, 1977).

Inability to Recognize Faces

The ability to recognize faces is also predominantly a right hemisphere function. The left hemisphere can select one face from a group only if an outstanding characteristic of the target face can be verbally represented, such as a moustache or glasses. People with right hemisphere lesions have great difficulty recognizing pictures of famous people in magazines or newspapers. Some patients cannot even recognize their own close relatives. One patient of mine never spoke first in any social interchange. He admitted that he could not recognize anyone, not even his wife, by facial appearance, but rather, he identified people by their voices. This failure to recognize faces has been called prosopagnosia.

Other Symptoms

Some patients with right hemisphere lesions have difficulty sustaining a muscular contraction, particularly keeping their eyes closed (Joynt et al., 1962). This deficit—called motor impersistence—may be due to the impairment of a cerebral mechanism for gauging kinesthetic feedback from contracting muscles (Carmon, 1970).

Many patients with right hemisphere lesions have abnormal postures. They are slouched in wheelchairs, or seemingly stuffed in one portion of the bed. Attempts to improve their uncomfortable positions are only transiently successful. This abnormal posture is not due solely to weakness, since it is not seen with right hemiplegia.

Most patients with right cerebral disease have some degree of emotional flattening. They may speak in a monotone, without emphasis or inflection, or even without any affective qualities (Ross and Mesulam, 1979). They also may have difficulty recognizing the emotional tone in the speech of others (Tucker et al; 1977).

EVALUATION

When he approaches the patient suspected of right hemisphere dysfunction, the physician must be alert to his own behavior as well as the patient's. He observes the patient's dress, posture, and appearance, but refrains from any remark about an obvious hemiplegia. Beginning the interview with noncommittal questions, he attempts to gauge the patient's knowledge of his own left side. The physician must keep a poker face no matter how seemingly outrageous are the patient's comments.

Commonly encountered is the patient who knows he has a weak side and spontaneously comments on it, but has no concern over this disability. He may refer to his left arm as though it did not belong to him. "This arm here," he says pointing but not looking at it, "doesn't seem to want to work." Less common, but still not infrequent, is the patient who has been told he is hemiplegic and has no reason to doubt medical authority, but really doesn't believe it.

Patient: They say I had a stroke.

Examiner: How did it affect you?

Patient: They say my arm can't move.

Much less common is the patient who actually denies his hemiplegia. This is not the vehement denial of the overwhelmed person who cannot accept a catastrophic loss. Rather, the patient is bland, perhaps slightly puzzled. While not really euphoric, he seems a bit amused by the suggestion that his left arm is paralyzed. The patient may react to the examiner's prodding to move his left arm in many ways. He may move his right arm; he may move his hemiplegic arm with his good hand; he may report that he doesn't want to move his arm right. The rarest patient is the one who not only denies his weakness, but actually denies his arm. His left arm belongs to someone else, perhaps the examiner, perhaps some unidentified person who is sharing his hospital bed. In general, this syndrome develops suddenly from loss of brain tissue, usually by stroke or by sacrifice of normal tissue during operation. The natural course is one of improvement. Rarely and always very transiently, denial of right hemiplegia (associated with aphasia) can be seen in a left hemisphere lesion in a right-handed person.

I recently saw a patient who identified his own arm held before his face as the examiner's arm but recognized his own wristwatch; he was at a loss to explain how his wristwatch had gotten on the doctor's wrist. My most unusual right hemisphere case was a patient who asked to see me after his first night in the hospital. He said he understood that veterans' hospitals had to cut corners financially but putting two patients in the same bed was too much. His left side felt so foreign to him that he thought another person was in the bed with him.

The patient with a right hemisphere lesion, even a longstanding one, will probably have difficulty drawing figures and geometric designs. The patient who is asked to copy simple figures or to draw a flower or clock will often plead lack of ability. Gentle persistence, tempered with emphasis on the routine nature of the examination, should counter this declination. The drawing of a clock will sometimes be so small that hardly anything can be seen. If the examiner draws the outline of the clock and asks the patient to draw in numbers and hands, there often results an opening spiral of numbers which begins normally but drifts across the page. A typical example is shown in Figure 2.

A patient's abilities with maps can be tested by asking him to draw one. The average person, however, may never have drawn a map and his attempts will show it. He has certainly seen and consulted many maps, however, and the examiner can himself draw a map and ask the patient to point out prominent points. I draw the continental United States and ask the patient to point out Florida, California, and New York. Most normal people in this location can draw the typical oblong outline of Tennessee in the southeast portion of a U.S. map outline.

Some neurologists keep a series of pictures of famous people to test facial recognition, such as U.S. Presidents. Most physicians will find such a collection burdensome because of infrequent use. When faced with a patient with suspected right hemisphere dysfunction, one can usually find lying about a magazine or newspaper containing a photograph or political cartoon depicting a well known political, sports, or entertainment personality. When showing the picture to the patient, one must be careful to exclude written identifying material.

Based upon these and other tests summarized in Table 1, the physician decides if a right hemisphere lesion is present. While this syndrome diagnosis

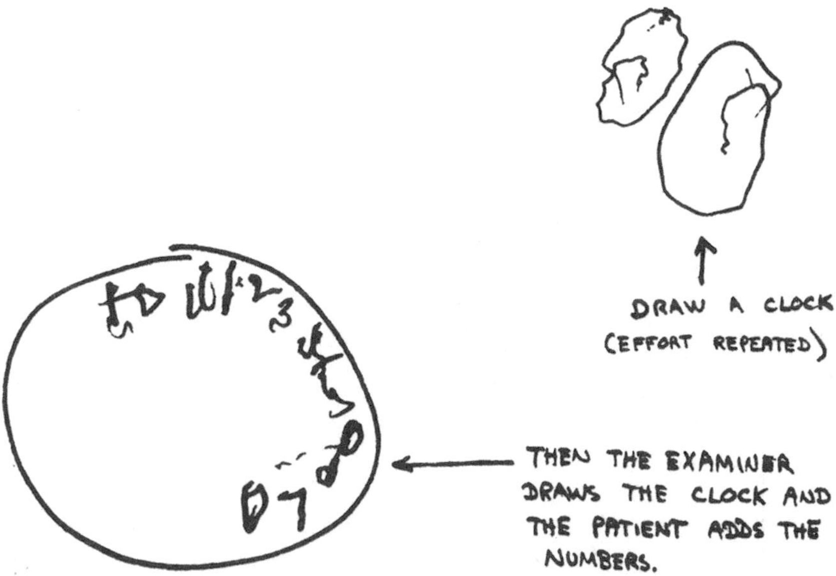

Figure 2: Another patient with a right hemisphere lesion has difficulty drawing a clock. When he puts numbers on a clock drawn by the examiner he fails to use the left portion of the circle.

is usually easy, borderline decisions are based upon mild dysfunction in all these abilities.

PATHOPHYSIOLOGY

The term aphasia denotes the major (but not all) symptoms that follow a left hemisphere lesion. The disorder of spatial orientation and body image that accompanies right hemisphere dysfunction has no analogous inclusive term. Suggestions include unilateral spatial agnosia (Caltagirone et al., 1977), spatial neglect (Chedru, 1976), and hemi-inattention (Weinstein and Friedland, 1977). Hughlings Jackson's original term—imperception—might be the best.

The aphasia produced by a lesion in the anterior portion of the left hemisphere differs from the aphasia produced by a posterior lesion. No clear analogous anterior to posterior differentiation of right hemisphere symptomatology is possible, although the full range of symptoms usually occurs only with posterior lesions. While hemi-inattention can be produced by frontal lesions, it is much more commonly a result of parietal destruction (Rosenberger, 1974). Frontal lesions seldom, if ever, produce constructional

Table 1: Major Deficits Following Right Hemisphere Lesions

Dysfunction	*Pedantic Term*	*Bedside Demonstration*
Denial of hemiplegia	Anosognosia	Noncommittal questions about medical history
Denial of left side	Hemisomatognosia	Patient asked to identify his own left hand
Disregard of left space	Hemi-inattention	Double simultaneous stimulation, line bisection
Impaired design abilities	Constructional apraxia	Draw or copy common geometrical figures
Inability to read maps	Acartagnosia	Patient points to major features on outline map
Cannot maintain muscle contraction	Motor impersistence	Ask patient to keep eyes closed
Inability to recognize faces	Prosopagnosia	Patient identifies pictures of prominent persons
Inability to dress properly	Dressing apraxia	Observe patient's appearance

apraxia, while parietal ones almost always do (McFie, 1969). The full right hemisphere disorder can be produced by a thalamic as well as a cortical lesion (Watson and Heilman, 1979), which is not surprising considering the thalamocortical interrelationships reviewed in Chapter 2. The greatest trouble recognizing faces results from a lesion at the right temporal occipital junction, usually combined with a left hemisphere lesion (Meadows, 1974). Cohn and co-workers conclude that bilateral destruction of the temporal fusiform gyrus produces prosopagnosia or as they put it, "the consolidation of visually related immediate memory, with particular reference to the human face, is resident in the fusiform gyri."

Animal studies have shown that limbic and brain stem lesions can produce some elements of hemi-inattention. Destruction of the cingulate gyrus (Watson, 1973) or the lateral mesencephalic reticular formation (Watson, 1978) produces a monkey who does not pay full attention to a touch on the contralateral side of his body. These studies lead to suggestions that most aspects of the right hemisphere syndrome result from a predominant problem of poor attention (Heilman and Watson, 1977) or flattened emotionality (Heilman et al., 1978).

Kinsbourne (1977) conceives each hemisphere responsible for orientation to the opposite half-world. Normally in balance, the destruction of one leads to an overpowering tendency of the remaining hemisphere to attend to contralateral activities. The greater spatial abilities concentrated in the right hemisphere (perhaps relegated there by a left hemisphere with special language responsibilities), cause greater hemi-inattention following right hemisphere destruction.

It seems that we are a long way from understanding right hemisphere pathophysiology. The clinical observations are real but cannot be explained.

IMPORTANCE

Neuropsychological signs and symptoms associated with right hemisphere lesions possess localizing value. Imagine a patient with vague complaints of left arm or leg weakness; general examination is normal except for a left Babinski sign. More detailed evaluation might indicate constructional apraxia and other signs of right hemisphere involvement, sparing the patient unnecessary diagnostic tests such as myelography or electromyography. A patient with a weak right arm could have peripheral nerve or spinal cord disease, but not if he also suffers the typical aphasic language deficits of left hemisphere dysfunction. Similarly, the occurrence of right hemisphere neuropsychological symptoms in a patient with complaints about his left side can point the clinician to appropriate evaluation for focal brain disease. The physician with a knowledge of minor hemisphere function has an additional diagnostic ability that can prevent unnecessary discomfort and expense to his patients.

The patient and his family can benefit from counseling. Even simple suggestions can sometimes be immensely helpful. Relatives who experience difficulty communicating with the recent stroke patient may be sitting on the patient's inattentive side; communication will be markedly improved by the simple expedient of moving their chairs. When the patient goes home, predictions about what to expect can allay concern. The patient who cannot find his own bathroom is not crazy or hopelessly demented; he is suffering from a predicted brain dysfunction which should improve with time. The patient should probably not drive a car until full recovery has occured, since he may have difficulty sensing vehicles approaching him from his left. Therapy for hemi-inattention, analogous to speech therapy, has been attempted but the only reported series had no control group; its results were confounded by the natural improvement in this condition (Diller and Weinberg, 1977).

The evaluation discussed in this chapter takes only a few minutes, much less than the time it takes to read about them, and can be intriguing when abnormalities are discovered. The attribution of these deficits to the right hemisphere can lead to appropriate etiologic diagnosis and therapy. Appreciation of minor hemisphere pathophysiology by the physician permits counseling that can aid the patient and his family in understanding and overcoming these disabilities.

Chapter 11

Temporal Lobe Epilepsy

EPILEPSY

In the last century, Hughlings Jackson defined a seizure as a change in behavior due to an abnormal paroxysmal discharge of cerebral gray matter. Buttressed by subsequent scientific developments such as electroencephalography, this definition excludes other episodic conditions, such as ordinary panic or anger, or the sleep attacks of narcolepsy. Lay people frequently disregard this rather restrictive medical definition and call any unexpected event a seizure, e.g., a myocardial infarction is a "heart seizure."

A seizure is a reaction of the brain to certain pathological circumstances. Seizures characterize certain types of metabolic disruptions, as discussed in the chapter on delirium. While all people can seize under appropriate metabolic stress, some individuals have such a low threshold that they experience seizures at any time. The tendency to recurrent seizures is called epilepsy. It should be noted that some restrict the term epilepsy to recurrent seizures of undefinable etiology.

While the predominant symptomatology of most seizures involves intense muscular movements, some seizures are characterized by psychic phenomena. These have been called the psychic equivalent of epilepsy, or thought seizures. While these old terms are occasionally revived (especially in the popular literature), most physicians today use the interchangeable terms psychomotor or temporal lobe seizures (Janovic, 1974). Neither term is ideal, however, since sometimes psychomotor seizures have no motor component, and temporal lobe seizures can be produced from a discharging focus in the frontal lobe or the cingulate gyrus (Geier et al., 1976). An international committee advanced the tongue twister partial seizures with complex symptomatology or, for short, complex partial seizures (Penry and Daly, 1975). This chapter will use the somewhat older but more widely recognized terms.

CLINICAL SYMPTOMATOLOGY

The typical psychomotor seizure begins with an unusual feeling or sensation. This heralding event—considered to be a warning by the patient—is actually part of the seizure, being produced by Jackson's paroxysmal discharge of gray matter. This first part of the seizure, which can occur alone, is called the aura, a term from an original case of Galen's who felt a breeze on his arm preceding a seizure. Videotape studies show that the initial observable change in the patient's behavior is a stare (Escueta et al., 1977). The stare is associated with a motionless frozen posture lasting from two to 10 seconds. The patient then develops automatic, repetitive motions like chewing, blinking, stomping the feet, picking at clothing. This behavior, called the automatism, lasts a further 10 to 60 seconds and fades into a period of confusion. The patient wanders about and can interact with his environment, but is amnestic for events occurring in this final stage, which can last for several minutes.

The clinical symptomatology is so diverse that the "typical" case described in textbooks contains elements from many actual patients. The novice diagnostician is frequently misserved by the textbook amalgam; the patient under consideration could not suffer temporal lobe epilepsy, he reasons, since he has only a small minority of the listed symptoms. Since there is no real "typical" case, let me summarize four recent patients from my own practice.

Case 1: A 28-year-old man had great difficulty describing his seizures. Sometimes they began with a rather unpleasant taste and smell and a feeling something like thick saliva in the mouth. The patient was then tongue-tied for just a few seconds. One prominent spell occurred as he was ordering food in a cafeteria; the serving person became impatient as he tried to communicate what he wanted; he was not even able to point. As the months went by, the character of the aura or warning changed; now a visual distortion heralded the spell. These were especially common in the shower; it seemed like the colored flowers on the shower curtain assumed a strange appearance with a change in their coloring.

During his physical examination, a seizure occurred. His face went slack while his jaws dropped open. He raised his hand, saying, "uh . . . uh . . . uh," not looking at the examiner. In five or ten seconds he was normal, specifically volunteering that he had had one of his spells.

An EEG showed somewhat equivocal left temporal epileptiform activity (Figure 1). A CT scan showed a temporal lobe tumor which, upon removal, proved to be a malignant glioma (Figure 2).

Case 2: A 20-year-old man had experienced unusual smells since the age of

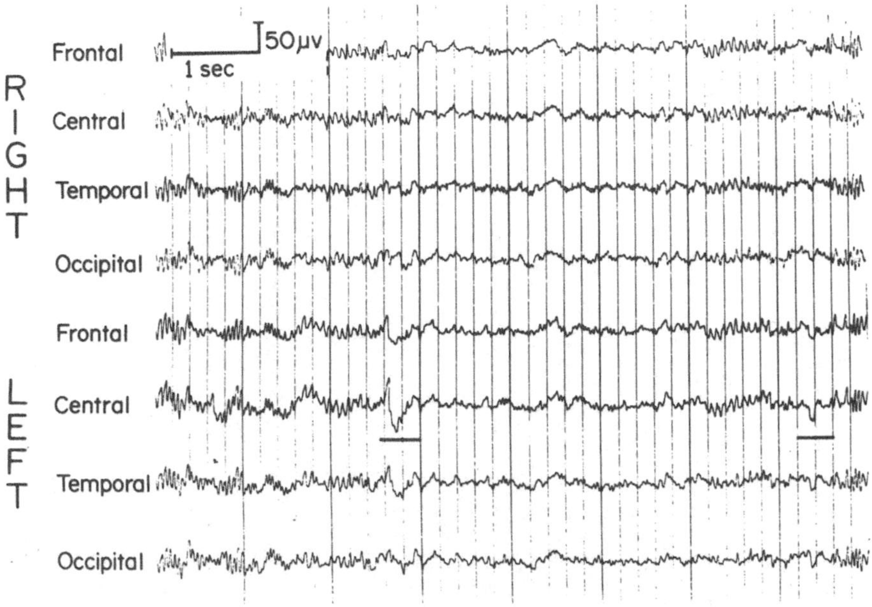

Figure 1: A 28-year-old man with strange spells has a suspicious discharge recorded by the EEG.

12. They were pleasant smells, almost indescribably so. When pushed for a comparison he suggested a flower, "but not like any earthly flower." The smells were not followed by unusual behavior or feelings but on other occasions he had very strong sensations of dejà vu. Since these smells and feelings had not bothered him he never told a physician about them.

One day, while on service with the U.S. Army, he began acting strangely; walking about, mumbling, doing inexplicable things like sitting in a sink full of dirty dishes. The next day at the hospital, he was amnestic for this behavior, in fact for almost the entire day.

The man's EEG showed right temporal epileptiform activity. The remainder of his evaluation was normal and he returned to limited duty, without driving or working at heights, under anticonvulsant therapy. No etiology could be delineated.

Case 3: A 43-year-old man had suffered a shotgun blast to his head in an altercation with a (former) friend several years previously. Shotgun pellets penetrated the skull and also destroyed his right eye. For many years thereafter, the patient had unusual spells where he thought someone was approaching him from the left. The identity of this person (who was never seen or heard, just felt) varied with the situation. One time, he was sitting on

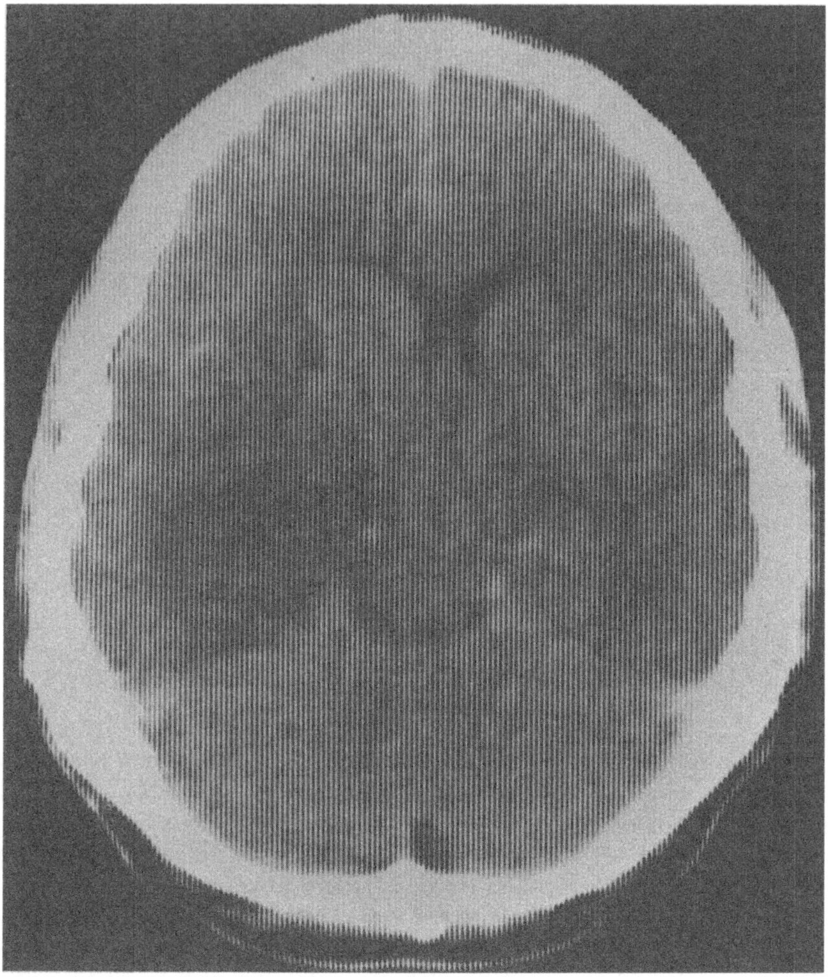

Figure 2: An unenhanced CT shows a large tumor. The patient's neurological and mental status examinations were normal despite the large size of this infiltrating glioma (case 1).

the porch watching his child in the front yard. Despite the fact that he could see his child, he could not shake the feeling that the very same child was out of his vision to his left. He frequently turned his head and eyes to reassure himself nothing was there. On another occasion, he stopped his car on the road because he had the hallucinated feeling that someone he knew was following just behind him. People who had observed him while he had these strange feelings reported that they were not accompanied nor followed by any change in behavior.

The patient did not seek any help for these spells and only came to medical attention when he had a nocturnal major motor seizure. The patient's wife heard gurgling sounds one night. Turning on the light she saw her husband develop bed-shaking, tonic-clonic movements with urinary incontinence. He was totally amnestic for this nocturnal seizure.

The EEG showed right temporal slowing, mixed with epileptiform sharp waves. Etiology of the seizure disorder was gliosis subsequent to direct brain trauma.

Case 4: A 48-year-old man developed spells beginning with an unpleasant smell. His mouth then filled with saliva. He thought that the saliva itself was malodorous and had forced his relatives to admit they experienced the odor, but they really didn't. The spell then proceeded to a strange feeling (described only as dizziness) and a change in vision, characterized by objects getting smaller or larger. When watching television, for example, one half the screen might seem to come closer while the other half receded.

The patient experienced these spells almost daily for several months. He mentioned them to his personal physician but no specific evaluation or treatment was undertaken. A routine chest x-ray showed a lung mass and a pulmonary specialist obtained neurological consultation for what he thought were transient ischemic attacks. Subsequent workup disclosed lung cancer metastatic to right temporal lobe.

SYNDROME DIAGNOSIS

The first step in diagnosis is to determine if the patient's spells are psychomotor seizures. The differential diagnosis of spells characterized by amnesia has been considered in Chapter 7. The key to diagnosis is detailed description. The patient provides an account of his subjective experience; no one else can describe the aura. It is absolutely imperative to obtain a description of the patient's behavior from another observer, even if the patient thinks his behavior was normal. This observer, usually the spouse, was probably quite frightened, perhaps even panicky, during the seizure, but her description as obtained by a trained interviewer is certainly closer to actual events than the patient's second-hand repetition of what others have told him.

Differentiation of psychomotor seizures from other episodic disorders, such as transient ischemic attacks or the absences of petit mal epilepsy, is based upon the character of the aura and the details of the behavior during the automatism (Dreifuss, 1975). The aura is characterized by strangeness, an ineffable feeling, an indescribable smell. Some elements of dejà vu are common among the general population (Richardson and Winokur,

1967), but a strong feeling of familiarity followed by automatic behavior provides important information for the diagnosis of psychomotor seizures. Occasionally, retrograde amnesia erases the memory of the aura; the spouse reports that the patient comments about an unusual odor before his automatism, but the patient has no memory for this smell. The characteristic behavior during the seizure can be quite different from patient to patient. Some behaviors involve the mouth with chewing movements or slobbering. Some repetitious movements give their names to the disorder as though they deserved separate classification, such as running, laughing, or crying epilepsy.

A common diagnostic problem involves differentiating epileptic rage from ordinary anger. While the visible evidence of anger almost always begins suddenly, when the perpetrator "just can't take it anymore" and hurls a breakable object against the wall, the feeling of anger builds up over several minutes or even hours. True epileptic rage is extremely rare, while ordinary anger is common, perhaps even universal. The attribution of violence to epileptics, either during or between seizures, is so misunderstood that a section of this chapter is devoted to this supposed association.

A rare patient has limbic or temporal lobe discharge occurring so often that his mental state does not return to normal between psychomotor seizures. This state of prolonged confusion may be mistaken for dementia. Usually this patient with psychomotor status has an hour-by-hour variation in mental status examination (Engel et al., 1978). Diagnosis is important because long term anticonvulsant therapy can significantly improve mental function and social life. One patient underwent 30 psychiatric hospitalizations before the correct diagnosis was made (Adebimpe, 1977).

The EEG is the only laboratory test of value for the syndrome diagnosis of temporal lobe epilepsy. Since the EEG only samples about an hour of real time, the recording of a clinical seizure is too much to hope for, unless the patient's seizures recur so frequently that his condition approaches status epilepticus. Fortunately, most epileptic individuals show isolated sharp waves and spikes in the EEG between clinical seizures (Figure 3). This interictal activity is not associated with any clinical change in the patient's behavior (thus not fulfilling Jackson's definition of a seizure), but has a similar appearance to the more prolonged discharge which does accompany a clinical seizure. Hence, this abnormality is termed epileptiform and its occurrence is utilized as corroborative evidence for the syndrome diagnosis of temporal lobe epilepsy. Neurons in a human epileptic focus discharge in disorganized bursts; when this burst activity spreads to adjacent neurons, an epileptiform spike is recorded by the overlying scalp electrodes (Babb and Crandall, 1976). A completely normal EEG should not deter diagnosis if descriptions of the spells are sufficiently characteristic; it is possible that the hour of recording time simply falls between interictal epileptiform waves.

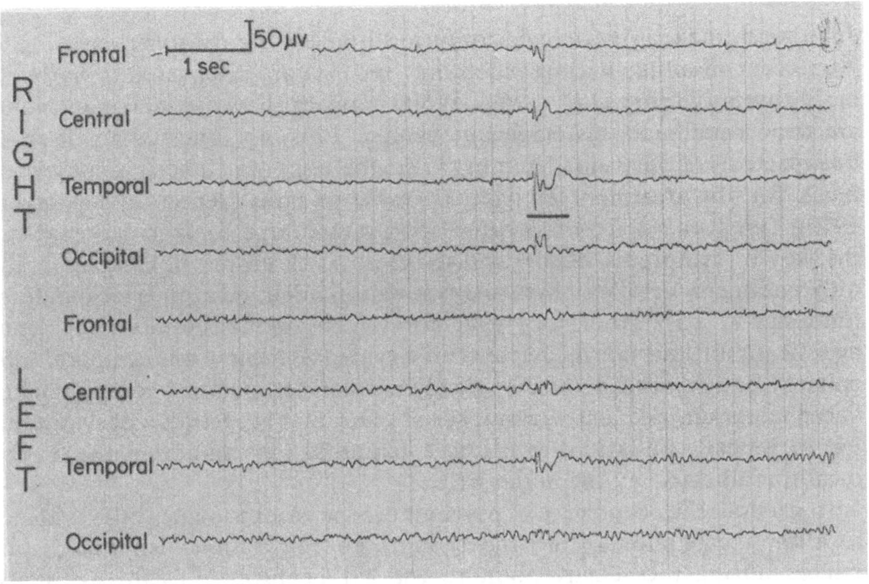

Figure 3: An unequivocal epileptiform discharge is recorded from a 20-year-old soldier (case 2).

Various methods have been advanced in order to bring out these interictal abnormalities, the two most common being nasopharyngeal electrodes to sample the electrical activity of medial brain structures, and sleep. Very frequently, epileptiform activity occurs only after a patient falls asleep, for reasons not at all clear (Freemon, 1978). If a patient with vague spells has a normal EEG, the knowledgeable physician will wonder if this was entirely recorded in the waking state.

ETIOLOGIC DIAGNOSIS

Once the syndrome diagnosis has been made, the physician can proceed to a consideration of etiology. Head trauma is a frequent cause of temporal lobe seizures, because of the vulnerability of the temporal lobe to collision with the bony borders of the middle fossa, as discussed in Chapter 7. Apparently, medial temporal structures are very sensitive to anoxia and an epileptogenic lesion can be produced by a wide variety of hypoxic events—from extraction difficulty at the time of birth, to a prolonged major motor seizure with cyanosis.

In the search for etiology, the physician emphasizes those entities amenable to specific treatment. While one must not overlook the rare case of seizures secondary to recurrent hypoglycemia or other episodic metabolic disruption, the major etiologic concern is brain tumor. In some series, up to 20 percent of adults with psychomotor seizures are discovered to harbor a brain tumor (Carney et al., 1969). While many of these are malignant, some are very small and histologically benign. It is not unusual to discover unexpectedly a very small tumor when the temporal lobe is removed en block for the treatment of uncontrollable seizures (Jensen and Klinken, 1976). Temporal lobe tumors can reach a rather large size and cause little in the way of symptoms besides the seizures. As discussed in Chapter 3, the only finding on detailed physical examination might be a superior quadrantanopsia. A past laboratory evaluation with normal results is evidence against tumor, but not incontrovertible evidence. I know one temporal lobe epilepsy patient who had a completely normal isotope brain scan, pneumoencephalogram, and arteriogram; seven years later progression of symptoms led to repeat evaluation, revealing a temporal lobe tumor in the precise location indicated by the initial EEG.

In general, the occurrence of psychomotor seizures provides little evidence to allow localization of the underlying lesion. Sometimes, aphasic disturbances during the seizure point to the left hemisphere as in case 1 just related. If the patient recalls elements of the automatism and if the automatic or forced movements include turning of the eyes and head, the clinician can suspect that the epileptic focus involves nontemporal portions of the limbic system such as orbitofrontal or cingulate cortex (Geier et al., 1976). The best known relationship of aura to neuroanatomical structure relates the uncus to the perception of an odor. This relationship was first noted by Jackson with his physician patient known as Queran and has been corroborated many times (Daly, 1958). Efforts to utilize psychomotor seizures to map emotional relationships in the temporal lobe the way Jackson mapped the precentral gyrus from the study of focal motor seizures have been largely unsuccessful (see, for example, King and Ajmone Marsan, 1977).

Remillard and his co-workers (1977) have found an asymmetry of facial movement with emotional stimulation in psychomotor epileptics. The side of the decreased movement is contralateral to the involved temporal lobe. In stroke patients with obvious hemiplegia, the facial weakness can be overcome by emotion, especially by laughing, presumably because of limbic input to the facial nucleus. I test for this when on teaching rounds by announcing that the senior resident and I have just developed a new diagnostic test. First the resident relates one of his corny jokes, I say, and the patient laughs politely, using voluntary input to the facial nucleus and demonstrating obvious asymmetry. Then I tell one of my hilarious jokes and every neuron in the patient's brain reverberates with mirth, overcoming the weakness. The people observing laugh as does the patient, and usually his weakness disappears just as predicted. Remillard and co-workers (1977) describe the opposite phenomenon; the cortex and basal ganglia are intact but the limbic system is not. Therefore, voluntary facial movement is normal, but emotion induces a clear asymmetry.

VIOLENCE

Popular authors from Dostoevski to Crichton have attributed to epileptics a special proclivity to bursts of uncontrollable violence. Surveys have found a higher incidence of epilepsy among prison inmates, especially those convicted of assault, than among the general populace, but the reasons for this are unclear. In the words of Lewis (1975), "those who hit other people on the head in bars are likely to be hit back and the occurrence of EEG foci or clinical seizures is likely to be much higher" than in a control population.

The phenomenon of undirected rage occurring during a temporal lobe seizure, although very rare, probably does exist. Many cases have been reported; most attacks appear to have some relationship to alcohol ingestion (Marinacci, 1963; Thompson, 1963). I have only encountered one individual who might represent an instance of this syndrome. This middle-aged man had experienced three separate instances of this characteristic behavior over a period of years: after having just two or three drinks in a bar he attacked a complete stranger, professing amnesia for the attack and the events leading up to it, recalling only entering the bar and "awakening" in the police station. He was not undergoing any court proceedings at the time he consulted me and seemed truly anxious to understand his puzzling behavior. A waking and sleeping EEG were normal, but after he drank a small amount of liquor clear epileptiform discharges were recorded from temporal leads. He had no clinical or emotional concomitants to these electrical abnormalities, no anger, no memory difficulty, and the giant bruiser of an orderly I had the foresight to station nearby was never needed. He had no further attacks on anticonvulsant therapy.

The reluctance of a court to punish a person for an act he cannot remember, combined with the tendency of an obviously guilty defendant to grasp at straws, have produced some ludicrous trials. Some "experts" argued that the Oswald murder, shown on live television, was the product of an epileptic seizure. The full transcript of this trial has been published in the medical literature in order to illustrate one of those rare occasions when lawyers show more common sense than doctors (State v. Jack Ruby, 1964).

While epileptic violence is rare, a physician often must consider it. For example, a teenager, known to have suffered epilepsy for many years, broke a glass pane in a door in the schoolyard during what the teachers called epileptic rage. She was not allowed to return to school until her doctors guaranteed against recurrence. One of my colleagues, believing the adage "when in doubt, take a history," went to the schoolyard and interviewed other children who had seen the attack in question. Actually, it was revealed, the girl had fallen backward and smashed the door with her body during the tonic-clonic phase of a major motor seizure. No rage was involved in this or any of her hundreds of previous fits, so the physicians gave the stupid "guarantee" required by the school authorities.

In my experience most epileptics who are labelled violent have reacted to attempts to hold them down during a seizure. Imagine yourself awakening as from sleep with four or five strangers holding you tightly on a dissecting table. You can't quite catch the words, but two of these strangers are mumbling something to each other about "trying further injections." Suppose you weren't quite able to talk, but could groan and struggle. I am sure you would not be surprised to find your actions described as combative. If all the strangers were members of a different race, your struggles might be even more strained. The physician who encounters a patient in a state of postictal confusion should not force him into a combative role; rather, he should explain briefly but repeatedly where the patient is and what has happened. He should guide him rather than force him to a position of safety.

BEHAVIORAL DISORDER

Many clinicians have observed that some temporal lobe epileptics have odd personalities. A personality, like a face, is hard to describe and it has not been easy to specify what exactly is unusual about this subgroup of patients. From her review of the literature, Stevens (1975) drew up this list of adjectives, each advanced by one or more authors to illustrate the "typical" psychomotor epileptic:

> adhesive, aggressive, apathetic, antagonistic, ambitious, bigoted, brutal, circumstantial, compulsive, depressed, dissatisfied, dyscontrolled, dysphoric, egocentric, emotional, explosive, fickle, garrulous, hypersexual, hyperactive, hypergraphic, hyposexual, hostile, inadequate, impulsive, importunate, irritable, litiginous, meticulous, moody, monotonous, narrow-minded, obstinate, paranoid, pedantic, peevish, perseverative, rage-prone, retarded, religious, slow, shy, sensitive, schizoid, shallow, sticky, stubborn, suspicious, temperamental, viscous, withdrawn, and willful.

Nonsense like this has led many investigators to conclude that the so-called "psychomotor epileptic personality" is just another myth about epilepsy akin to the violence myth.

Many attempts to delineate abnormal personality traits have utilized formal psychological testing. Every conceivable standardized test, from large personality inventories like the MMPI to projective tests like the Rorschach, have failed to differentiate psychomotor epilepsy patients from other epileptics or even from normals (Small et al., 1962; Stevens et al., 1972). Unusual individual patients or small groups of patients, such as the epileptics who wrote long, philosophical, rambling essays (Waxman and Geschwind, 1974), were felt to represent highly selected instances culled from a large referral practice.

Bear and Fedio (1977), utilizing a special test of their own design, clearly differentiated psychomotor epileptics as a group from normal individuals and from nonepileptic patients. They developed 100 sentences which they thought might characterize the odd personality described in the clinical literature. Each patient (and his spouse) indicated if a particular sentence applied to him. (For example the trait circumstantiality was represented by the sentence: "I have trouble getting to the point because of all the details.") The temporal lobe epileptics experienced more intense emotions, both euphoria and sadness, than the nonepileptic control groups. They were more hostile, angry, and self-recriminatory. They were religious, moralistic, and humorless. They overinterpreted motives and events to the point of paranoia. They had pathological degrees of organization, orderliness, and compulsive attention to detail, with extensive diaries and notes. They complained of feeling helpless at the hands of fate. Of special interest were the different responses of those patients with a left temporal EEG focus from those patients with a right temporal discharge. The patients with seizures originating from the left temporal lobe showed more anger, more paranoia, a greater sense of helplessness, and a greater sense of the personalized significance of events. Those with right temporal discharging foci showed more emotion, sadness and euphoria, as well as a greater compulsive attention to detail.

In evaluating the interesting results of Bear and Fedio (1977), it is important to note that their patients suffered seizures for a very long time, ranging between six and 35 years, with an average of almost 20. Not all patients with temporal lobe epilepsy show these behavioral characteristics. None were present in any of the four cases presented earlier in this chapter, for example. Those patients showing odd personalities are often those who have had the most seizures over the longest period of time.

This leads to the concept of hyperconnection, advanced by Bear and Fedio (1977) to explain these behavioral quirks. The concept seems a bit fanciful, but it may represent a new form of neurological dysfunction and, therefore, bears examination. Cutting pathways between two brain areas can produce a dysconnection syndrome, as discussed in Chapter 9; perhaps excessive seizure discharge along a seldom-used pathway can connect (hyperconnect) disparate brain regions. In behavioral terms, perhaps the temporal association between a mundane event and the deep emotion of an epileptic aura produces a confused meaning about the importance of the event. The patient might overinterpret environmental occurrences, might feel incapable of controlling his feelings, and/or might feel a pawn in the hands of higher powers. Another explanation for the odd personalities of some psychomotor epileptics supposes that underlying damage to the limbic system produces both seizures and personality disorders. Kristensen and Sindrup (1978) found that psychomotor epileptics with paranoid ideation attributed to psychosis had a greater amount of brain damage by many different criteria than did psychomotor epileptics without psychiatric symptomatology.

If these behavioral characteristics do occur in psychomotor epileptics, it would not be too surprising to find an occasional patient whose symptoms became so severe as to influence his judgement. So-called "epileptic psychosis," the conjoining of psychotic thinking and epilepsy, results. Flor-Henry (1969) made the interesting observation that institutionalized patients with left temporal epileptic foci were more frequently diagnosed as schizophrenic, while right temporal lobe epileptics more frequently received the diagnosis of manic-depressive psychosis. The findings of Bear and Fedio (1977) explain this diagnostic variation; left temporal foci are more frequently associated with paranoia, right temporal with emotional changes—both euphoria and depression.

To summarize, an interictal behavioral disorder does exist in some patients with temporal lobe epilepsy, especially those with many years of seizures. In a very rare patient, the disorder can become so severe that a diagnosis of functional psychosis can be made. Waxman and Geschwind (1975) feel that the personality disorder can be so characteristic that it can provide evidence for the syndrome diagnosis of temporal lobe epilepsy.

TREATMENT

As with other neuromental disorders described in this book, treatment of the patient with psychomotor seizures is aimed at both etiology and syndrome, and counseling is one of the most important functions of the physician. Only a minority of patients will have an underlying etiology amenable to specific medical or surgical therapy.

The mainstay of therapy for the syndrome of recurrent psychomotor seizures involves long-term pharmacological treatment (Table 1). Most clinicians in the United States begin therapy with phenytoin (formerly called diphenylhydantoin), while most in Europe begin with carbamazepine. American physicians are wary of the hematological side effects, especially because of a special warning required by the Food and Drug Administration. European physicians accept the rather frequent, but transient decrease in blood count and the very rare fatal bone marrow suppression of carbamazepine, in order to escape the mild, but bothersome mental effects of phenytoin. Phenytoin's depression of intellectual function is so mild that it is usually not clinically evident, and can be appreciated only by crossover studies comparing psychological and clinical effects of phenytoin and carbamazepine (Troupin et al., 1977). An advantage of phenytoin over carbamazepine is its longer half-life; in most patients, phenytoin can be given twice or even once per day, while carbamazepine's more rapid metabolism dictates its administration at least thrice daily.

Counseling involves three points:

1) an attempt to explain the basis of the seizure;
2) a delineation of how the disorder limits the patient's activities;
3) emphasis on the importance of taking the anticonvulsant medication regularly.

The first of these points is extremely difficult. One analogy relates the epileptic focus to a short circuit in an electrical machine, emphasizing how much of the patient's life is completely normal with only a rare "short circuit overload." I had a good counseling session with a patient one day; the next morning I read about the patient's suicide. The reader may be wise to take advice on counseling from someone else (for example, Rodin, 1975). Simply let me warn you that many patients, even some from high socio-economic backgrounds, harbor subconscious thoughts about epilepsy which seem to hark back to primitive times.

One must warn the patient of his limitations; he should avoid situations where a loss of consciousness might lead to disaster, such as working at heights, swimming alone, and especially driving a vehicle. The counselor should emphasize all the things a patient can do. Some physicians forbid contact sports, from fears about head injuries aggravating the seizure disorder, but such advice places the patient in an invalid role from which he may never recover. Because severe alcohol abuse definitely worsens (or perhaps even creates) seizure disorder, some physicians forbid their epileptic patients the social use of alcohol. Such advice may unnecessarily stigmatize an individual whose life is already severely restricted.

The behavior disorder associated with longstanding temporal lobe epilepsy is treated like any other behavior disorder. If the patient's mental world is disrupted by disabling paranoia or thought disorder, he often benefits from pharmacological treatment with antipsychotic medication. Haloperidol is probably superior to the phenothiazines, because of the tendency of the latter to increase seizure frequency.

The key to seizure control is the maintenance of a therapeutic serum level of one or more anticonvulsant drugs. While metabolism varies with the individual, the greatest variation in serum level devolves from the percentage of the prescribed medicine ingested (Blackwell, 1973). This is called patient

TABLE 1: Anticonvulsants Commonly Used for the Treatment of Temporal Lobe Epilepsy

Generic Name	*Major Trade Name*	*Average Oral Dosage Per Day*	*Therapeutic Serum Level*	*Reference*
Phenytoin	Dilantin	400 mg	15 μg/ml	Lund, 1974
Carbamazepine	Tegretol	1200 mg	4 μg/ml	Monaco et al., 1976
Phenobarbital	many	300 mg	25 μg/ml	Dreifuss, 1979
Primidone	Mysoline	1000 mg	5 μg/ml	Kutt and Penry, 1974
Valproic acid	Depakene	2000 mg	50 μg/ml	Bruni and Wilder, 1979

compliance (the patient complies with the physician's wishes); the patient probably calls it physician communication. If the serum level is zero when the patient's dose of phenytoin is 300 mg per day, little value accrues from raising the prescribed dosage; if the patient does not take three tablets, he will probably also not take four. The physician should confront the patient with the paradox and emphasize that with this type of long-term condition the patient is a partner in his own medical care; actually he is the partner with the controlling interest.

To be complete the surgical treatment of temporal lobe epilepsy should be mentioned. If the seizures cannot be controlled with anticonvulsant medication, and if the EEG indicates that the abnormal activity is originating from one temporal lobe, then surgical removal of the epileptogenic lesion can be indicated. Other surgical approaches are in the experimental stage and are mainly applied to major motor or grand mal seizures; these include certain stereotaxic lesions of the motor system (Yoshii, 1978) and chronic electrical stimulation of the cerebellum (Cooper and Upton, 1978), as well as corpus callosal section as discussed in Chapter 2.

Chapter 12

Epilogue

I hope that this short book has given the reader the flavor of organic mental disease, and a glimpse of the fascination and exasperation of working with these patients, who are poorly served by modern medicine. "The unfortunate patient's malfunctioning brain rests in limbo," said Engel and Romano (1959), "an object of interest neither to the medical man nor to the psychiatrist" and the only thing that has changed in 20 years is the term "medical man."

As I see the future, the plight of these patients worsens. Psychiatry seems to be moving away from brain disorders. Some futurologists have even predicted that psychiatry as an entity will disappear, plunging into a void between clinical psychology, which will aid with problems of living, and neurology, which will treat true diseases like schizophrenia (Torrey, 1978). But neurology is not ready to take on these traditional psychiatric disorders; in fact, as I view the contemporary scene, neurology is edging away from organic mental disease patients. For example, virtually every advertisement for a practicing neurologist announces a requirement for expertise in electromyography.

One psychiatrist has predicted that not only will psychiatry fade away, but it will be accompanied by all of medicine. The physician will be replaced by a hospital corpsman who will feed a patient's history and physical findings into a nearby computer, which will order the appropriate laboratory tests (just the appropriate ones), then give diagnosis and prescribe therapy. "Because a medic-computer symbiosis will usurp all the tasks presently assigned to physicians, doctors will be rendered obsolete" (Maxmen, 1976). Don't you think that some of the patients described in this book would make the medic-computer sympiosis weep?

The personal interaction between doctor and patient, the gathering of clinical data, the formulation of a management plan, is the most important but least emphasized cog in the health care production line. How much research funding goes to study the clinical (not laboratory) diagnostic process? This interaction is the least reimbursable physician activity under existing insurance programs, leading physicians to more remunerative procedures such as, for the neurologist, electromyography. The change from private to government control magnifies the problem. For example, the first decade of the Canadian government health care system saw the time spent in each physician-patient interaction drop by 60 percent (Mueller, 1978).

Putting aside these theoretical musings, and returning to the unending war against disease, the physician approaches the battle against organic mental disease with almost an empty arsenal. Technological backup hurts as often as it helps. The physician seems to stand alone on the bridge, armed only with his abilities and his knowledge. I hope your knowledge has been honed and your morale raised by this brief book.

You are now ready for the most complex and recalcitrant organic mental disease patient. Here is an example, related by Dr. Samuel Shem (1978):

> The hairy-armed nurse told Potts that the woman on the stretcher was his first admission of the day, named Ina Goober. Ina was a great mass of flesh sitting upright on a stretcher, wearing, like a uniform, a gown that had blazoned across its front, "The New Masada Nursing Home." Glowering, Ina clutched her purse. She was yelling a high pitched GO AVAY GO AVAY GO AVAY . . .
>
> Potts did what the textbooks [like this one?] said to do: introduced himself, saying, "Hello, Mrs. Goober, I'm Dr. Potts. I'll be taking care of you."
>
> Upping her volume, Ina screamed: GO AVAY GO AVAY GO AVAY . . .
>
> Potts next tried to engage her using the other textbook method, grasping her right hand. Quick as lightning Ina struck him a southpaw blow with her purse, knocking him back against the counter.

So, put this book down, take a deep breath, and re-enter the fray. Mrs. Ina Goober and thousands like her are waiting for you.

References

Abler WL: Asymmetry in the skulls of fossil man: evidence of lateralized brain function? *Brain Behav Evol 13:* 111–115, 1976.

Abuzzahab FS Sr, Merwin GE, Zimmerman RL et al.: A double blind investigation of piracetam (Nootropil) vs placebo in geriatric memory. *Pharmakopsychiat 10:* 49–56, 1977.

Adebimpe VR: Complex partial seizures simulating schizophrenia. *J Amer Med Ass 237:* 1339–1341, 1977.

Alajouanine T: Aphasia and artistic realization. *Brain 74:* 299–241, 1948.

Albert ML, Feldman RG, Willis AL: The "subcortical dementia" of progressive supranuclear palsy. *J Neurol Neurosurg Psychiat 37:* 121–130, 1974.

Albert MS, Butters N, Levin J: Temporal gradients in the retrograde amnesia of patients with alcoholic Korsakoff's disease. *Arch Neurol 36:* 211–216, 1979.

Alkar GJ Jr, Glasauer FE, Leslie EV: Long-term experience with isotope cisternography. *J Amer Med Ass 219:* 1005–1010, 1972.

Allen GI, Tsukahara N: Cerebrocerebellar communication systems. *Physiol Rev 54:* 957–1006, 1974.

Allen RM, Young JJ: Phencyclidine-induced psychosis. *Amer J Psychiat 135:* 1081–1084, 1978.

Allison RS, Hurwitz LJ: On perseveration in aphasics. *Brain 90:* 429–448, 1967.

Amadeo M, Roemer RA, Shagass C: Can callosal speed of transmission be inferred from verbal reaction times? *Biol Psychiat 12:* 289–297, 1977.

April RS, Tse PC: Crossed aphasia in a Chinese bilingual dextral. *Arch Neurol 34:* 766–770, 1977.

Arieff AI, Cooper JD, Armstrong D et al.: Dementia, renal failure, and brain aluminum. *Ann Int Med 90:* 741–747, 1979.

Asanuma H, Hunsperger RW: Functional significance of projection from the cerebellar nuclei to the motor cortex in the cat. *Brain Res 98:* 73–92, 1975.

Asokan SK, Vansant J, Bassett WB et al.: Delayed recognition of lead encephalopathy in two "moonshine" drinkers. *Southern Med J 67:* 1440–1442, 1974.

Babb TL, Crandall PH: Epileptogenesis of human limbic neurons in psychomotor epileptics. *Electroencephal Clin Neurophysiol 40:* 225–243, 1976.

Babinski JF: Contribution a l'etude des troubles mentaux dans l'hemiplegie organique cerebrale (anosognosie). *Rev Neurol 22:* 845–848, 1914. Reprinted in DA Rottenberg and FH Hochberg (eds.) *Neurological Classic in Modern Translation*, Hafner Press, 131–135, 1977.

Bakan P, Dibb G, Reed P: Handedness and birth stress. *Neuropsychol 11:* 363–366, 1973.

Banta RG, Markesbery WR: Elevated manganese levels associated with dementia and extrapyramidal signs. *Neurology 27:* 213–216, 1977.

Barr AN, Heinze WJ, Dobben GD et al.: Bicaudate index in computerized tomography of Huntington disease and cerebral atrophy. *Neurology 28:* 1196–1200, 1978.

Barr AN, Heinze W, Mednoze JE et al.: Long-term treatment of Huntington disease with glutamate and pyriodoxine. *Neurology 28:* 1280–1282, 1978.

Barrett-Conner E: The etiology of pellagra and its significance for modern medicine. *Amer J Med 42:* 859–867, 1967.

Battersby WS, Bender MB, Pollack M et al.: Unilateral spatial agnosia (inattention) in patients with cerebral lesions. *Brain 93:* 68–93, 1956.
Bear DM, Fedio P: Quantitative analysis of interictal behavior in temporal lobe epilepsy. *Arch Neurol 34:* 454–467, 1977.
Becker GC, Davis JL, Parell GJ: Pseudocaloric nystagmus. *Arch Neurol 35:* 93–94, 1978.
Bender MB: Single episode of confusion with amnesia. *Bull NY Acad Med 36:* 197–207, 1960.
Bennett JA, Trinder J: Hemispheric laterality and cognitive style associated with transcendental meditation. *Psychophysiol 14:* 293–296, 1977.
Benson DF: Amnesia. *Southern Med J 71:* 1221–1228, 1978.
Benson DF, Marsden CD, Meadows JC: The amnesic syndrome of posterior cerebral artery occlusion. *Acta Neurol Scandinav 50:* 133–145, 1974.
Benson DF, Sheremata WA, Bouchard R et al.: Conduction aphasia: a clinicopathological study. *Arch Neurol 28:* 339–346, 1973.
Benton AL: Historical notes on cerebral dominance. *Arch Neurol 34:* 127–129, 1977.
Benton AL, Levin HS, Varney NR: Tactile perception of direction in normal subjects: implications for hemispheric cerebral dominance. *Neurology 23:* 1248–1250, 1973.
Benton AL, Varney NR, Hamsher K de D: Lateral differences in tactile directional perception. *Neuropsychol 16:* 109–114, 1978.
Berlin CI, Hughes LF, Lowe-Bell SS: et al.: Dichotic right ear advantage in children 5 to 13. *Cortex 9:* 393–401, 1973.
Berlucchi G, Heron W, Hyman R et al.: Simple reaction times of ipsilateral and contralateral hand to lateralized visual stimuli. *Brain 94:* 419–430, 1971.
Bernstein S, Leff R: Toxic psychosis from sleeping medicines containing scopolamine. *N Engl J Med 277:* 638–639, 1967.
Betts TA, Smith WT, Kelly RE: Adult metachromatic leukodystrophy (sulphatide lipidosis) simulating acute schizophrenia. *Neurology 18:* 1140–1142, 1968.
Bever TG, Chiarello RJ: Cerebral dominance in musicians and non-musicians. *Science 185:* 537–539, 1974.
Bickerstaff ER: *Neurological Examination in Clinical Practice.* Blackwell, Oxford, 1973, p. 9.
Birkett DP, Boltuch B: Measuring dementia. *J Amer Geriat Soc 25:* 153–156, 1977.
Black PM: Criteria of brain death: review and comparison. *Postgrad Med J 57:* 69–74, 1975.
Black D, Woollacott S: Acute toxic psychosis in two children treated with benzhexol hydrochloride (Artane). *Brit J Psychiat 125:* 483–484, 1974.
Blackburn IW: *Gross Morbid Anatomy of the Brain in the Insane.* Govt Printing Off. Washington, D.C., 1908.
Blackwell G: Drug therapy. *N Engl J Med 289:* 249–252, 1973.
Blass JP, Gibson GE: Abnormality of a thiamine-requiring enzyme in patients with Wernicke-Korsakoff syndrome. *N Engl J Med 297:* 1367–1370, 1977.
Blocker WW Jr, Kastl AJ Jr, Daroff RB: Psychiatric manifestations of cerebral malaria. *Amer J Psychiat 125:* 192–196, 1968.
Bogen JE, Bogen GM: Wernicke's region: Where is it? *Ann NY Acad Aci 280:* 834–843, 1976.
Borst CV, ed.: *The Mind-Brain Identity Theory.* Macmillan, New York, 1970.
Bosch EP, Hart MN: Late adult-onset metachromatic leukodystrophy. *Arch Neurol 35:* 475–477, 1978.
Botez ML, Ethier R, Leveille J et al.: A syndrome of early recognition of occult hydrocephalus and cerebral atrophy. *Quart J Med 46:* 365–380, 1977.
Botez ML, Fontaine F, Botez T et al.: Folate-responsive neurological and mental disorders: Report of 16 cases. *Eur Neurol 16:* 230–246, 1977.
Brandt KD, Cohen AS: Cerebral disorders of vision in systemic lupus erythematous. *Ann Int Med 83:* 163–169, 1975.
Brendler SJ, Selverstone B: Recovery from decerebration. *Brain 93:* 381–392, 1970.

Brenner I: Bromism: alive in well. *Amer J Psychiat 135:* 857–858, 1978.

Brewer C: Psychosis due to acute hypothyroidism during the administration of carbimazole. *Brit J Psychiat 115:* 1181–1183, 1969.

Brice DD, Hetherington RR, Utting JE: A simple study of awareness and dreaming during anaesthesia. *Brit J Anaesth 42:* 535–542, 1970.

Brodal A: *Neurological Anatomy: Its Relation to Clinical Medicine.* 2nd ed., Oxford University Press, New York, 1969.

Brown DG, Goldensohn ES: The electroencephalogram in normal pressure hydrocephalus. *Arch Neurol 29:* 70–71, 1973.

Brownell GL, Correia JA, Hoop B Jr: Scintillation scanning of the brain. *Ann Rev Biophys Bioeng 3:* 365–386, 1974.

Bruni J, Wilder BJ: Valproic acid: Review of a new antiepileptic drug. *Arch Neurol 36*: 393–398, 1979.

Buchanan DC, Abram HS: Psychotic behavior resulting from a lateral ventricle meningioma: A case report. *Dis Nerv Syst 36:* 400–401, 1975.

Bucy PC, Keplinger JE, Siqueira EB: Destruction of the "pyramidal tract" in man. *J Neurosurg 21:* 385–398, 1964.

Burns HS, Lerner SE: Perspectives in acute phencyclidine intoxication. *Clin Toxicol 9:* 477–501, 1976.

Bursten B: On not talking with patients: A message to the new medical student. *Pharos 42:* 18–20, 1978.

Butler RN: Alzheimer's disease, senile dementia and related disorders: The role of NIA. In *Alzheimer's Disease*, Katzman R, Terry RD, and Bick KL, (eds.) Raven Press, New York, 1978.

Byrd GJ: Acute organic brain syndrome associated with gentamicin therapy. *J Amer Med Ass* 53–54, 1977.

Cairns H, Oldfield RC, Pennybacker JB et al.: Akinetic mutism with an epidermoid cyst of the third ventricle. *Brain 64:* 273–290, 1941.

Caltagirone C, Micelli G, Gainotti G: Distinctive features of unilateral spatial agnosia in right and left brain damaged patients. *Eur Neurol 16:* 121–126, 1977.

Caplan LR, Hedley-White T: Curing and memory dysfunction in alexia without agraphia: a case report. *Brain 97:* 251–262, 1974.

Caplan LR, Schoene WC: Clinical features of subcortical arteriosclerotic dementia (Binswanger disease). *Neurology 28:* 1206–1215, 1978.

Capote B, Parikh N (1978) Cyclandelate in the treatment of senility: a controlled study. *J Amer Geriat Soc 26:* 360–362, 1978.

Carlen PL, Wortzman G, Hogate RC et al.: Reversible cerebral atrophy in recently abstinent chronic alcoholics measured by computed tomography scans. *Science 200:* 1076–1078, 1978.

Carmon A: Impaired utilization of kinesthetic feedback in right hemisphere lesions. *Neurology 20:* 1033–1038, 1970.

Carmon A, Harishanu Y, Lowinger E et al.: Asymmetries in hemispheric blood volume and cerebral dominance. *Behav Biol 7:* 853–859, 1972.

Carmon A, Nachson I: Ear asymmetry in perception of emotional non-verbal stimuli. *Acta Psychol 37:* 351–357, 1973.

Carney LR, Hudgins RL, Espinosa RE et al.: Seizures beginning after the age of 60. *Arch Intern Med 124:* 707–709, 1969.

Celesia CG: Pathophysiology of periodic EEG complexes in subacute sclerosing panencephalitis (SSPE). *Electroenceph Clin Neurophysiol 35:* 293–300, 1973.

Celesia GG, Barr AN: Psychosis and other psychiatric manifestations of levodopa therapy. *Arch Neurol 23:* 193–200, 1970.

Chambers JF, Schultz JD: Double-blind study of three drugs in the treatment of acute alcoholic states. *Quant J Stud Alcoh 26:* 10–18, 1965.
Chapman LF, Wolff HG: The cerebral hemispheres and the highest integrative functions in man. *Arch Neurol 1:* 357–424, 1959.
Chartock HE, Glassman PR, Poon LW et al.: Changes in alpha rhyth, during learning of verbal and visuospatial tasks. *Physiol Behav 15:* 237–239, 1975.
Chatrain CE, White LE Jr, Shaw CM: EEG pattern resembling wakefulness in unresponsive decerebrate state following traumatic brain stem infarct. *Electroenceph Clin Neurophysiol 16*: 285–289, 1964.
Chedru F: Space representation in unilateral spatial neglect. *J Neurol Neurosurg Psychiat 39:* 1057–1061, 1976.
Chierchetti SM, Ferrari P, Sala P et al.: Effects of amantidine on mental status of elderly patients: a double-blind comparison with placebo. *Curr Therap Res 22:* 158–165, 1977.
Cherington M: Visual neglect in a chess player. *J Nerv Ment Dis 159:* 145–147, 1974.
Cherington M, Ott JE, Robinson A: Cornelia de Lange syndrome in an adult male. *Neurology 19:* 879–884, 1969.
Ch'ien LT, Boehm RM, Robinson H et al.: Characteristic early electroencephalographic changes in herpes simplex encephalitis. *Arch Neruol 34:* 361–364, 1977.
Clark EO, Glanzer M, Turndorf H: The pattern of memory loss resulting from intravenously administered diazepam. *Arch Neurol 36:* 296–300, 1979.
Clark JA, Davidson LJ, Ferguson HC: Psychosis in hypoparathyroidism. *J Ment Sci 108:* 811–815, 1962.
Cohen DN, Salanga VA, Hully W et al.: Alexia with agraphia. *Neurology 26:* 455–459, 1976.
Cohen SI, Marks IM: Prolonged organic psychosis with recovery in Addison's disease. *J Neurol Neurosurg Psychiat 24:* 366–368, 1961.
Cohn R, Neumann MA, Wood DH: Prospagnosia: a clinicipathologic study. *Ann Neurol 1:* 177–182, 1977.
Cooper IS, Upton ARM: Use of chronic cerebellar stimulation for disorders of disinhibition. *Lancet 1:* 595–600, 1978.
Coren S, Kaplan CP: Patterns of ocular dominance. *Amer J Optomet 50:* 283–292, 1973.
Coren S, Porac C: Fifty centuries of right-handedness: the historical record. *Science 198:* 631–632, 1977.
Corsellis JAN, Bruton CJ, Freeman-Browne D: The aftermath of boxing. *Psychol Med 3:* 270–303, 1973.
Corsellis JAN, Goldberg GJ, Norton AR: "Limbic encephalitis" and its association with carcinoma. *Brain 91:* 481–498, 1968.
Cranefield PF: *The Way In and the Way Out*. Futura Pubs, Mt. Kisco, New York, 1974.
Critchley M: Dr. Samuel Johnson's aphasia. *Med Hist 6:* 27–44, 1962.
Critchley M: The enigma of Gerstmann's syndrome. *Brain 89:* 183–198, 1966.
Croft PB, Heathfield KWG, Swash M: Differential diagnosis of transient amnesia. *Brit Med J 4:* 593–596, 1973.
Crook T, Ferris S, Sathananthan G: The effect of methylphenidate on test performance in the cognitively impaired aged. *Psychopharmacol 52:* 215–255, 1977.
Cross HE, McKusick VA: The Mast syndrome. *Arch Neurol 16:* 1–13, 1967.
Crowell RM, Tew JM, Mark VH: Aggressive dementia associated with normal pressure hydrocephalus. *Neurology 23:* 461–464, 1973.
Daly D: Uncinate fits. *Neurology 8:* 250–260, 1958.
Daly DD, Love JG: Akinetic mutism. *Neurology 8:* 238–242, 1958.
Davidson RJ, Schwartz GE: The influence of musical training on patterns of EEG asymmetry during musical and non-muscial self-generation tasks. *Psychophysiol 14:* 58–63, 1977.
Davies P, Maloney AJR: Selective loss of central cholinergic neurons in Alzheimer's disease. *Lancet 2:* 1403, 1976.

Davis LE, Wands JR, Weiss SA et al.: Central nervous system intoxication from mercurous chloride laxatives. *Arch Neurol 30:* 428–431, 1974.

DeJong RN: The hippocampus and its role in memory: Clinical manifestations and theoretical considerations. *J Neurol Sci 19:* 73–83, 1973.

DeLand FH, James AE Jr, Ladd DJ et al.: Normal pressure hydrocephalus. *Amer J Clin Pathol 58:* 58–63, 1972.

Denny-Brown D: Neurological conditions resulting from prolonged and severe dietary restriction. *Medicine 26:* 41–113, 1947.

Denny-Brown D: The nature of apraxia. *J Nerv Ment Dis 126:* 9–32, 1958.

Dewberry FL, McKinney TD, Stone WJ et al.: The dialysis dementia syndrome: report of ten cases and review of the literature. In press.

Diller L, Weinberg JP: Hemi-inattention in rehabilitation: The evolution of a rational remediation program. *Adv Neurol 18:* 63–82, 1977.

Dilts SL, Keleher DL, Hoge G et al.: Hydroxyzine in the treatment of alcohol withdrawal. *Amer J Psychiat 134:* 92–93, 1977.

Dimond SJ: *The Double Brain*, Chruchill Livingstone, Edinburgh, 1972.

Dimond S, Beaumont G: Hemisphere function and paired-associated learning. *Brit J Psychol 65:* 275–278, 1974.

Dinsdale H, Logue V, Piercy H: A case of persisting impairment of recent memory following right temporal lobectomy. *Neuropsychol 1:* 287–298, 1964.

Di Rocco C, DiTrapani G, Maira G et al.: Anatomo-clinical correlations in normotensive hydrocephalus. *J Neurol Sci 33:* 437–452, 1977.

Doktor R, Bloom DM: Selective lateralization of cognitive style related to occupation as determined by EEG alpha asymmetry. *Psychophyiol 14:* 385–387, 1977.

Donald AG, Still CN, Pearson JM: Behavioral symptoms with intracranial neoplasm. *Southern Med J 65:* 1006–1009, 1972.

Doose H, Volzke E: Dementia and petit mal. *Neuropediatrie 10:* 10–14, 1979.

Doyle JC, Ornstein R, Galin D: Lateral specialization of cognitive mode II: EEG frequency analysis. *Psychophysiol 11:* 567–578, 1974.

Drachman DA: Memory and cognitive function in man: Does the cholinergic system have a specific role? *Neurology 27:* 783–790, 1977.

Dreifuss FE: The differential diagnosis of partial seizures with complex symptomatology. *Adv Neurol 11:* 187–200, 1975.

Dreifuss FE: Use of anticonvulsant drugs. *J Amer Med Ass 241:* 607–609, 1979.

Dressler DM, Folk J: The treatment of depression with ECT in the presence of brain tumor. *Amer J Psychiat 132:* 1320–1321, 1975.

Dumas R, Morgan A: EEG Asymmetry as a function of occupation, task, and task difficulty. *Neuropsychol 13:* 219–228, 1975.

Ehyai AB, Fenichel GM: The natural history of acute confusional migraine. *Arch Neurol 35:* 368–369, 1978.

Ellis WG, McCulloch JR, Corley CL: Presenile dementia in Down's syndrome: ultrastructural identity with Alzheimer's disease. *Neurology 24:* 101–106, 1974.

Engel GL, Roman J: Delirium, a syndrome of cerebral insufficiency. *J Chron Dis 9:* 260–277, 1959.

Engel J, Ludwig BI, Fetell M: Prolonged partial complex status epilepticus: EEG and Behavioral observations. *Neurology 28:* 863–869, 1978.

Escueta AV, Kunze U, Waddell G: Lapse of consciousness and automatisms in temporal lobe epilepsy: a videotape analysis. *Neurology 27:* 144–155, 1977.

Fahn S, Craddock G, Kremin G: Acute toxic psychosis from suicidal overdosage of amantadine. *Arch Neurol 25:* 45–48, 1971.

Favazza AR, Martin P: Chemotherapy of delirium tremens: a survey of physician's preferences. *Amer J Psychiat 131:* 1031–1033, 1974.

Feigl H: *The Mental and the Physical.* U Minn Press, Minneapolis, 1967.
Feinstein AR: *Clinical Judgement.* Williams and Wilkins, Baltimore, 1967.
Feldman RG, Chandler KA, Levy LL et al.: Familial Alzheimer's disease. *Neurology 13:* 811–824, 1963.
Ferraro A, Arieti S, English WH: Cerebral changes in the course of pernicious anemia and their relationship to psychic syndromes. *J Neuropath Exp Neurol 4:* 217–239, 1945.
Filbey RA, Gazzaniga MS: Splitting the normal brain with reaction time. *Psychonom Sci 12:* 335–338, 1969.
Fincham RW, Nibbelink DW, Aschenbrener CA: Alexia with left homonymous hemianopsia without agraphia: a case report with autopsy findings. *Neurology 25:* 1164–1168, 1975.
Fisher CM: The neurological examination of the comatose patient. *Acta Neurol Scandinav Supp 36:* 1–56, 1969.
Fisher CM, Adams RD: Transient global amnesia. *Acta Neurol Scandinav 40, Suppl 9:* 1–83, 1964.
Flor WJ, Stevenson JS, Ghaed N et al.: Cisternograms in the primate Macaca mulatta. *Neurology 24:* 266–270, 1974.
Flor-Henry P: Schizophrenic-like reactions and affective psychoses associated with temporal lobe epilepsy: etiological factors. *Amer J Psychiat 126:* 400–403, 1969.
Foroozan P, Trier HS: Mucosa of the small intestine in pernicious anemia. *N Engl J Med 277:* 533–559, 1967.
Fox JH, Ramsey RG, Huckman MS et al.: Cerebral ventricular enlargement: chronic alcoholics examined by computerized tomography. *J Amer Med Ass 236:* 365–368, 1976.
Fox JH, Topel JL, Huckman MS: Use of computerized tomography in senile dementia. *J Neurol Neurosurg Psychiat 38:* 948–953, 1975.
Fox RH, Davies TW, Marsh FP et al.: Hypothermia in a young man with an anterior hypothalamic lesion. *Lancet 2:* 185–188, 1970.
Freeman JM, Finkelstein JD, Mudd SH: Folate-responsive homocystinuria and "schizophrenia": A defect in methylation due to deficient 5, 10-methylenetetrahydrofolate reductase activity. *N Engl J Med 292:* 491–496, 1975.
Freemon FR: Akinetic mutism and bilateral anterior cerebral artery occlusion. *J Neurol Neurosurg Psychiat 34:* 693–698, 1971.
Freemon FR: Oscar Wilde: poet, novelist, playwright, homosexual. *Med Aspects Human Sexuality 6:* 113–124, 1971.
Freemon FR: Evaluation of patients with progressive intellectual deterioration. *Arch Neurol 33:* 658–659, 1976.
Freemon FR: Two roads to coma. *Medical Hypothesis 2:* 82–84, 1976.
Freemon FR: Sleep in patients with organic disease of the nervous system. In Williams RW and Karacan I (eds.) *Diagnosis and Treatment of Sleep Disorders.* Wiley, New York, 1978.
Freemon FR, Douglas EFO, Penry JK: Environmental interaction and memory during petit mal (absence) seizures. *Pediatrics 51:* 911–918, 1973.
Freemon FR, Drake FT: Abnormal emotional reaction to hospitalization jeopardizing medical treatment. *Psychosom 8:* 150–155, 1967.
Freemon FR, Goodwin DW, Halikas JA, et al.: An electroencephalographic study of memory loss during alcoholic intoxication. *Dis Nerv Syst 32:* 848–852, 1971.
Freemon FR, McNew JJ, Adey WR: Sleep of unrestrained chimpanzee: cortical and subcortical recording. *Exp Neurol 25:* 129–137, 1969.
Freemon FR, Nevis AH: Temporal lobe sexual seizures. *Neurology 19:* 87–90, 1969.
Freemon FR, Walter RD: Electrical activity of human limbic system during sleep. *Comprehensive Psychiat 11:* 544–551, 1970.
French JD: Brain lesions associated with prolonged unconsciousness. *Arch Neurol Psychiat 68:* 727–740, 1952.

Friedberg J: Shock treatment, brain damage, and memory loss: a neurological perspective. *Amer J Psychiat 134:* 1010–1014, 1977.

Froeschels E: Is handedness organic or functional in nature? *Amer J Psychotherap 15:* 101–105, 1961.

Gaitz CM, Varner RV, Overall JE: Pharmacotherapy for organic brain syndrome in late life. *Arch Gen Psychiat 34:* 839–845, 1977.

Gajdusek DC, Gibbs CJ Jr, Asher DM et al.: Precautions in the medical care of, and in handling materials from, patients with transmissible virus dementia (Creutzfeldt-Jakob disease). *N Engl J Med 297:* 1253–1258, 1977.

Gascon G, Victorm D, Lombroso CT et al.: Language disorder, convulsive disorder, and electroencephalographic abnormalities: acquired syndrome in children. *Arch Neurol 28:* 156–162, 1973.

Gates A, Bradshaw JL: The role of the cerebral hemisphere in music. *Brain Lang 4:* 1–29, 1977.

Gazzaniga MS: *The Bisected Brain*, Appleton-Century-Crofts, New York, 1970.

Gazzaniga MS, Bogen JE, Sperry RW: Dyspraxia following division of the cerebral commissures. *Arch Neurol 16:* 606–612, 1967.

Gazzaniga MS, Freedman H: Observations on visual processes after posterior callousal section. *Neurology 23:* 1126–1130, 1973.

Gazzaniga MS, Sperry RW: Simultaneous double discrimination response following brain bisection. *Psychonom Sci 4:* 261–262, 1966.

Gazzaniga MS, Sperry RW: Language after section of the cerebral commissures. *Brain 90:* 131–148, 1967.

Geier S, Bancaud J, Talairach J et al.: Automatisms during frontal lobe epileptic seizures. *Brain 99:* 447–458, 1976.

Geschwind N: Aphasia. *N Engl J Med 284:* 654–656, 1971.

Geschwind N: Case 15–1975, differential diagnosis. *N Engl J Med 292:* 852–857, 1975.

Geschwind N: Anatomical asymmetry as the basis for cerebral dominance. *Fed Proc 37:* 2263–2266, 1978.

Geschwind N, Quadfasel FA, Segarra JM: Isolation of the speech area. *Neuropsychol 6:* 327–340, 1968.

Gerstmann J: Syndrome of finger agnosia, disorientation for right and left agraphia and acalculia. *Arch Neurol Psychiat 44:* 398–427, 1940.

Gilbert C, Bakan P: Visual asymmetry in perception of faces. *Neuropsychol 11:* 355–362, 1973.

Gilbert GJ: Quinidine dementia. *J Amer Med Ass 237:* 2093–2096, 1977.

Gilbert GJ: Transient global amnesia: manifestations of medial temporal lobe epilepsy. *Clin Electroenceph 9:* 147–152, 1978.

Gilbert JJ, Benson DF: Transient global amnesia: report of two cases with definite etiologies. *J Nerv Ment Dis 154:* 461–464, 1972.

Glass A, Butler SR: Alpha EEG asymmetry and speed of left hemisphere thinking. *Neurosci Lett 4:* 231–235, 1977.

Globus GG: Consciousness and the brain: the identity thesis. *Arch Gen Psychiat 29:* 153–160, 1973.

Gloning K: Handedness and aphasia. *Neuropsychol 15:* 355–358, 1977.

Go RCP, Todorov AB, Elston RC et al.: The malignancy of dementias. *Ann Neurol 3:* 559–561, 1978.

Goldfarb AI, Hochstadt JJ, Jacobsob JH: Hyperbaric oxygen treatment of organic mental syndrome in aged persons. *J Gerontol 27:* 212–217, 1972.

Goldstein LI: Emesis versus lavage for drug ingestion. *J Amer Med Ass 208:* 2162–2163, 1969.

Goldstein MN, Joynt RJ: Long-term follow-up of a callosal sectionized patient. *Arch Neurol 20:* 96–102, 1969.

Goodglass H, Kaplan E: Disturbance of gesture and pantomine in aphasia. *Brain 86:* 703–720, 1963.
Goodwin DW, Alderson P, Rosenthal R: Clinical significant of hallucinations in psychiatric disorders: a study of 116 hallucinatory patients. *Arch Gen Psychiat 24:* 76–86, 1971.
Goodwin DW, Othmer E, Halikas JA et al.: Loss of short-term memory as a predictor of the alcoholic "blackout". *Nature 227:* 201–202, 1970.
Goran A, Ciminello VJ, Fisher RG: Hemorrhage into meningiomas. *Arch Neurol 13*: 65–69, 1965.
Gordon HW, Bogen JE, Sperry RW: Absence of deconnection syndrome in two patients with partial section of the neocommissures. *Brain 94*: 327–336, 1971.
Gordon HW, Sperry RW: Lateralization of olfactory perception in the surgically separated hemispheres of man. *Neuropsychol 7:* 11–20, 1969.
Gorelick DA, Kussin SZ, Kahn I: Paranoid delusions and auditory hallucinations associated with digoxin intoxication. *J Nerv Ment Dis 166:* 817–819, 1978.
Green E, Howes DH: The nature of conduction aphasia: a study of anatomic and clinical features and underlying mechanisms. *Stud Neurolinguistics 3:* 123–156, 1977.
Greene HH, Bennett DR: Transient global amnesia with a previously unreported EEG abnormality. *Electroenceph Clin Neurophysiol 36:* 409–413, 1974.
Greenlee JE, Crampton RS, Miller JQ: Transient global amnesia associated with cardiac arrhythmia and digitalis intoxication. *Stroke 6:* 513–516, 1975.
Grozinger B, Kornhuber HH, Kriebel J: Methodological problems in the investigation of cerebral potentials preceding speech: determining the onset and suppressing artifacts caused by speech. *Neuropsychol 13:* 263–270, 1975.
Grundke-Iqbal I, Johnson AB, Wisniewski HM et al.: Evidence that Alzheimer neurofibrillary tangles originate from neurotubules. *Lancet 1:* 578–580, 1979.
Grunnet ML: Changing incidence, distribution, and histopathology of Wernicke's polioencephalopathy. *Neurology 19:* 1135–1139, 1969.
Guirguis EF: Management of disturbed patients: an alternative to the use of mechanical restraints. *J Clin Psychiat 39:* 295–303, 1978.
Gustafson L, Hagberg B: Recovery in hydrocephalus dementia after shunt operation. *J Neurol Neurosurg Psychiat 41:* 940–947, 1978.
Hachinski VC, Lasen NA, Marshall J: Multi-infarct dementia: a cause of mental deterioration in the elderly. *Lancet 2:* 207–210, 1974.
Hakim S, Adams RD: The special clinical problem of symptomatic hydrocephalus with normal cerebrospinal fluid pressure. *J Neurol Sci 2:* 307–327, 1965.
Hakola HPA, Iivanainen M: A new hereditary disease with progressive dementia and polycystic osteodysplasia: neuroradiological analysis of seven cases. *Neuroradiol 6:* 162–168, 1973.
Halgren E, Babb TL, Rausch R et al.: Neurons in the human basolateral amygdala and hippocampal formation do not respond to odors. *Neurosci Lett 4:* 331–335, 1977.
Harrison MJG, Marsden CD: Progressive intellectual deterioration (letter to the editor). *Arch Neurol 34:* 199, 1977.
Harrison MJG, Robert CM, Uttley D: Benign aqueduct stenosis in adult. *J Neurol Neurosurg Psychiat 37:* 1322–1328, 1974.
Hart MN, Cancilla PA, Frommes S et al.: Anterior horn cell degeneration and Bunina-type inclusions associated with dementia. *Acta Neuropath 38:* 225–228, 1977.
Hartley TC, Heilman KM, Garcia-Bengochea F: A case of a transient global amnesia due to a pituitary tumor. *Neurology 24:* 998–1000, 1974.
Hartmann A, Alberti E: Differentiation of communicating hydrocephalus and presenile dementia by continuous recording of cerebrospinal fluid pressure. *J Neurol Neurosurg Psychiat 40:* 630–640, 1977.
Hashi K, Nishimura S, Kondo A et al.: The EEG in normal pressure hydrocephalus. *Acta Neurochirur 33:* 23–35, 1976.

Havens LL: Taking a history from the difficult patient. *Lancet 1:* 138–140, 1978.
Hayward RW, Naeser MA, Zatz LM: Cranial computed tomography in aphasia: Correlation of anatomical lesions with functional deficits. *Radiology 123:* 653–660, 1977.
Heathfield KWG, Croft PB, Swash M: The syndrome of transient global amnesia. *Brain 96:* 729–736, 1973.
Heck AF, Hameroff SB, Hornick RB: Chronic Listeria monosytogenes meningitis and normotensive hydrocephalus. *Neurology 21:* 263–270, 1971.
Heffern PR, Pooro RS, Olson ME et al.: A demyelinating disorder associated with cerebrovascular amyloid angiography. *Arch Neurol 33:* 501–506, 1976.
Heilman KM: Ideational apraxia: a re-definition. *Brain 96:* 861–864, 1973.
Heilman KM, Fisher WR: Hyperlipidemic dementia. *Arch Neurol 31:* 67–68, 1974.
Heilman KM, Schwartz HD, Watson RT: Hypoarousal in patients with the neglect syndrome and emotional indifferences. *Neurology 28:* 229–232, 1978.
Heilman KM, Sypert GW: Korsakoff's syndrome resulting from bilateral fornix lesions. *Neurology 27:* 490–493, 1977.
Heilman KM, Valenstein E: Frontal lobe neglect in man. *Neurology 22:* 660–664, 1972.
Heilman KM, Watson RT: Mechanisms underlying the unilateral neglect syndrome. *Adv Neurol 18:* 93–106, 1977.
Heinz ER, Martinez J, Haenggeli A: Reversibility of cerebral atrophy in anorexia nervosa and Cushing's syndrome. *J Comp Assit Tomogr 1:* 415–418, 1977.
Heiser JF, Gillen JC: The reversal of anticholinergic drug-induced delirium and coma with physostigmine. *Amer J Psychiat 127:* 1050–1054, 1971.
Herbert V: Experimental nutritional folate deficiency in man. *Trans Assoc Amer Phys 75:* 307–320, 1962.
Herman M, Most H, Jolliffee N: Psychoses associated with pernicious anemia. *Arch Neurol Psychiat 38:* 348–361, 1937.
Hines D: Differences in tachisotscopic recognition between abstract and concrete words as a function of visual half-field and frequency. *Cortex 13:* 66–73, 1977.
Hirchkowitz M, Earle J, Paley B: EEG alpha asymmetry in musicians and non-musicians. a study of hemispheric specialization. *Neuropsychol 16:* 125–128, 1978.
Hodgins E: *Episode: Report on the Accident Inside My Skull.* Atheneum, New York, 1963.
Hoff J, Barber R: Transcerebral mantle pressure in normal pressure hydrocephalus. *Arch Neurol 31:* 101–105, 1974.
Hokfelt T, Ljungdahl A, Fuxe K et al.: Dopamine nerve terminals in the rat limbic cortex: aspects of the dopamine hypothesis of schizophrenia. *Science 184:* 177–179, 1974.
Hollender MH, Jamieson RC, McKee EA et al.: Anticholinergic delirium in a case of Munchausen syndrome. *Amer J Psychiat 135:* 1407–1409, 1978.
Hooshmand H, Sepdham T, Vries JK: Kluver-Bucy syndrome: successful treatment with carbamazepine. *J Amer Med Ass 229:* 1782, 1974.
Hughes CP, Myers FK, Smith K et al.: Nosologic problems in dementia. *Neurology 23:* 344–351, 1973.
Hunter R, Blackwood W, Bull J: Three cases of frontal meningiomas presenting psychiatrically. *Brit Med J 3:* 9–16, 1968.
Ignelzi RJ, Squire LR: Recovery from anterograde and retrograde amnesia after percutaneous drainage of a cystic craniopharyngioma. *J Neurol Neurosurg Psychiat 39:* 1231–1235, 1976.
Illingworth RD, Logue V, Symon L: The centriculocaval shunt in the treatment of adult hydrocephalus. *J Neurosurg 35:* 681–685, 1971.
Illis LS, Taylor FM: The electroencephalogram in herpes simplex encephalitis. *Lancet 1:* 718–721, 1972.
Ines DF, Markand ON: Epileptic seizures and abnormal electroencephalographic findings in hydrocephalus and their relation to the shunting procedures. *Electroceph Clin Neurophysiol 42:* 761–768, 1977.

Ingvár DH, Schwartz MS: Blood flow patterns induced in the dominant hemisphere by speech and reading. *Brain 97:* 273–288, 1974.

Iqbal K, Grundke-Iqbal I, Wisniewski HM et al.: Chemical relationship of the paired helical filaments of Alzheimer's dementia to normal human neurofilaments and neurotubules. *Brain Res 142:* 321–332, 1978.

Jacobs L, Conti D, Kinkel WR et al. "Normal pressure" hydrocephalus. *J Amer Med Ass 235:* 510–512, 1976.

Jaffe R. Bender MB: EEG studies in the syndrome of isolated episodes of confusion with amnesia. *J Neuro Neurosurg Psychiat 29:* 472–474, 1966.

Jarho L: Korsakoff-like amnesia syndrome in penetrating brain injury. *Acta Neurol Scandinav 49:* 19–156, 1973.

Jaynes J: *The Origin of Consciousness in the Breakdown of the Bicameral Mind.* Houghton Mifflin, Boston, 1977.

Jensen I, Klinken L: Temporal lobė epilepsy and neuropathology. *Acta Neurol Scandinav 54:* 391–414, 1976.

Jouvet M: Neurophysiology of the states of sleep. *Physiol Rev 47:* 117–177, 1967.

Jovanovic UJ: *Psychomotor Epilepsy: A Polydimensional Study.* Charles C. Thomas, Springfield, Illinois, 1974.

Kahn RL, Zarit SH, Hilbert NM et al.: Memory complaint and impairment in the aged. *Arch Gen Psychiat 32:* 1569–1573, 1975.

Kaim SC, Klett CJ, Rothfield B: Treatment of the acute withdrawal state: a comparison of four drugs. *Amer J Psychiat 125:* 1640–1646, 1969.

Karis R, Horenstein S: Localization of speech parameters by brain scan. *Neurology 26:* 226–230, 1976.

Kaszniak AW, Fox J, Gandell DL et al.: Predictors of mortality in presenile and senile dementia. *Ann Neurol 3:* 246–252, 1978.

Kataoka K, Sormachi M, Okuno S et al.: Cholinergic and gabaergic fibers in the stria medullaris of the rabbit. *Brain Res Bull 2:* 461–464, 1977.

Keddie KMG: Toxic psychosis following mumps. *Brit J Psychiat 111:* 691–696, 1965.

Killeffer FA, Stern WE.: Chronic effects of hypothalamic injury: report of a case of near total hypothalamic destruction resulting from removal of a craniopharyngioma. *Arch Neurol 22:* 419–429, 1970.

Kiloh LG, Gye RS, Rushworth RG et al.: Stereoactive amygdaloidotomy for aggressive behavior. *J Neurol Neurosurg Psychiat 37:* 437–444, 1974.

Kimura D: Functional asymmetry of the brain in dichotic listening. *Cortex 3:* 163–178, 1967.

King DW, Ajamone Marsan C: Clinical features and ictal patterns in epileptic patients with EEG temporal lobe foci. *Ann Neurol 2:* 138–147, 1977.

Kinsbourne M: Hemi-neglect and hemisphere rivalry. *Adv Neurol 18:* 41–50, 1977.

Kleist K: *Sensory Aphasia and Amusia.* Pergamon Press, New York, 1962.

Koranyi EK: Two cases of malaria presenting with psychiatric symptoms. *Biol Psychiat II:* 445–449, 1976.

Kreuter C, Kinsbourne M, Trevarthen C: Are deconnected cerebral hemispheres independent channels? A preliminary study of the effect of unilateral loading on bilateral finger tapping. *Neuropsychol 10:* 453–461, 1972.

Kristensen O, Sindrup EH: Psychomotor epilepsy and psychosis I: physical aspects. *Acta Neurol Scand 57:* 361–369, 1978.

Kutt H, Penry JK: Usefulness of blood levels of antiepileptic drugs. *Arch Neurol 31:* 283–288, 1974.

Lance JW: *The Mechanism and Management of Headache*, 2nd ed. Butterworth's, London, 1973, p. 10.

Langfitt TW: Measuring the outcome from head injuries. *J Neurosurg 48*: 673–678, 1978.

Laws ER, Mokri B: Occult hydrocephalus: results of shunting correlated with diagnostic tests. *Clin Neurosurg 24:* 316–333, 1977.

Leeks SR: A mid-brain lesion presenting as schizophrenia. *N Z Med J 66:* 311–314, 1967.

Leichnetz GR, Astruc J: Preliminary evidence for a direct projection of the prefrontal cortex to the hippocampus in the squirrel monkey. *Brain Behav Evol 11:* 355–364, 1975.

Lely AH, van Enter CHJ: Large-scale digitoxin intoxication. *Brit Med J 3:* 737–739, 1970.

Levine DN, Calvano R: A study of the visual defect in verbal alexia simultanagnosia. *Brain 101:* 65–81, 1978.

Levy J, Trevarthen C, Sperry RW: Perception of bilateral chimeric figures following hemisphere deconnection. *Brain 95:* 61–78, 1972.

Lewin K, Mattingly D, Millis RR: Anorexia nervosa associated with hypothalamic tumour. *Brit Med J 2:* 629–630, 1972.

Lewis C, Ballinger BR, Presly AS: Trial of levodopa in senile dementia. *Brit Med J 1:* 550–551, 1978.

Lewis JA: Violence and epilepsy. *J Amer Med Ass 232:* 1165–1167, 1975.

Lezak MD: *Neuropsychological Assessment.* Oxford University Press, New York, 1976.

Lichtheim L: On aphasia. *Brain 7:* 431–484, 1885.

Lindsley DB, Schreiner LH, Knowles WB et al.: Behavioral and EEG changes following chronic brain stem lesions in the car. *Electroenceph Clin Neurophysiol 2:* 483–498, 1950.

Lipowski ZJ: Delirium, clouding of consciousness and confusion. *J Nerv Ment Dis 145:* 227–255, 1967.

Lippold OCJ, Novotny GEK: Is alpha rhythm an artifact. *Lancet 1:* 976–979, 1970.

Lipton LM, Payne H, Garza HR et al.: Thermolability in Wernicke's encephalopathy. *Arch Neurol 35:* 750–753, 1978.

Liston EH Jr: Occult presenile dementia. *J Nerv Ment Dis 164:* 263–267, 1977.

Livingston KE, Escobar E: Anatomical bias of the limbic system concept: a proposed reorientation. *Arch Neurol 24:* 17–21, 1971.

Lizak RP, Zimmerman RA: Transient global amnesia due to a dominant hemisphere tumor. *Arch Neurol 34:* 317–318, 1977.

Locke S, Angevine JB, Yakovlev BI: Limbic nuclei of thalamic and connections of limbic cortex II: thalamocortical projection of the lateral dorsal nucleus in man. *Arch Neurol 4:* 355–364, 1961.

Loeb C, Rosadini G, Poggia GF: Electroencephalogram during coma: Normal and borderline records in five patients. *Neurology 9:* 610–618, 1959.

Lonnum A, Kornstad S: Long-term prognosis of patients with central cerebral ventricula enlargement. *Acta Neurol Scandinav 50:* 409–433, 1974.

Lopes de Silva FH, Storm van Leeuwen W: The cortical source of the alpha rhythm. *Neurosci Lett 6:* 237–241, 1977.

Lowe SS, Cullen JK, Berlin CI: Perception of simultaneous dichotic and monotic monosyllables. *J Speech Hearing Res 13:* 812–822, 1970.

Luessenhop AJ, Cruz TC, Fenichel GM: Surgical disconnection of the cerebral hemispheres for intractable seizures. *J Amer Med Ass 213:* 1630–1636, 1970.

Lund L: Anticonvulsant effect of diphenyldantoin relative to plasma levels. *Arch Neurol 31:* 289–294, 1974.

Luria AR, Tsvetkova LS, Futer JC: Aphasia in a composer. *J Neurol Sci 2:* 288–292, 1965.

MacLean PD: Psychosomatic disease and the "visceral brain": recent developments bearing on the Papez theory of emotion. *Psychosom Med 11:* 338–353, 1949.

MacLean PD: Some psychiatric implications of physiological studies on the frontotemporal portion of the limbic system (Visceral brain). *Electroenceph Clin Neurophysiol 4:* 407–418, 1952.

McAdam DW, Whittaker HA: Language production: electroencephalographic localization in the normal human brain. *Science 172:* 499–502, 1971.
McEntree WJ, Mair RG: Memory impairment in Korsakoff's psychosis: a correlation with brain noradrenergic activity. *Science 202:* 905–907, 1978.
McFie J: The diagnostic significance of disorders of higher nervous activity: syndrome related to frontal, temporal, parietal, and occipital lesions. In PJ Vinken, GW Bruyn (eds.), *Disorders of Higher Nervous Activity*, Vol. 4 of *Handbook of Clinical Neurology*, North Holland Publ. Co., Amsterdam, 1969.
McFie: *Assessment of Organic Intellectual Impairment*. Academic Press, New York, 1976.
McGeachie RE, Fleming JO, Sharer LR et al.: Diagnosis of Pick's disease by computed tomography. *J Comp Assist Tomogr 3:* 113–115, 1979.
McLeod SS, Peacock LJ: Tasks related EEG asymmetry: Effects of age and ability. *Psychophysiol 14:* 308–311, 1977.
McNealy DE, Plum F: Brainstem dysfunction with supratentorial mass lesions. *Arch Neurol 7:* 10–32, 1962.
Magnaes B: Communicating hydrocephalus in adults. *Neurology 28:* 478–484, 1978.
Magnes J, Moruzzi G, Pompeiano O: Synchronication of the EEG produced by low frequency electrical stimulation in the area of solitary tract. *Arch Ital Biol 99:* 33–67, 1961.
Magoun HW: The ascending reticular activating system and wakefulness. In JF Delafresnaye (ed.), *Brain Mechanisms and Consciousness*. Charles Thomas, Springfield, 1954.
Magoun HW: *The Waking Brain*, 2nd ed., Charles C. Thomas, Springfield, 1963.
Malamund N: Psychiatric disorder with intracranial tumors of limbic system. *Arch Neurol 17:* 113–123, 1967.
Manyam NVB, Hare TA, Katz L et al.: Huntington's disease: Cerebrospinal fluid GABA levels in at-risk individuals. *Arch Neurol 35:* 728–730, 1978.
Marinacci AA: A special type of temporal lobe (psychomotor) seizures following ingestion of alcohol. *Bull LA Neurol Soc 28:* 241–250, 1963.
Marino R Jr, Rasmussen T: Visual field changes after temporal lobectomy in man. *Neurology 18:* 825–835, 1968.
Marions O, Lying-Tunell U: Constancy of convexity air block on pneumoencephalography. *Neuroradiol 13:* 191–193, 1977.
Markand ON, Wheeler GL, Pollack SL: Complex partial status epilepticus (psychomotor status). *Neurology 28:* 189–196, 1978.
Marquardsen J, Harvald B: The electroencephalogram in acute vascular lesions of the brain stem and cerebellum. *Acta Neurol Scandinav 40:* 58–68, 1964.
Marsden CD, Harrison MJG: Outcome of investigation of patients with presenile dementia. *Brit J Med 2:* 249–252, 1972.
Martin JB: Neural regulation of growth hormone secretion. *N Engl J Med 288:* 1384–1393, 1973.
Martin JB, Banker BQ: Subacute multifocal leukoencephalopathy. *Arch Neurol 21:* 590–602, 1969.
Maruta T: Prescription drug-induced organic brain syndrome. *Amer J Psychiat 135:* 376–377, 1978.
Mateer C, Kimura D: Impairment of nonverbal oral movements in aphasia. *Brain Lang 4:* 262–276, 1977.
Matthews RA, Bookhammer RS, Izlar WH: Paresis: an analysis of 511 treated cases. *Amer J Psychiat 94:* 1259–1275, 1938.
Maxmen JS: *The Post-Physician Era*. Wiley, New York, 1976, p. 7.
Maxmen JS, Siberfarb PM, Ferrell RB: Anorexia nervosa: practical initial management in a general hospital. *J Amer Med Ass 229:* 801–803, 1974.
Mazza S, Laudisio A, Bergonzi P: Occult normal pressure hydrocephalus with parkinsonian symptomatology. *Eur Neurol 14:* 39–42, 1976.

Mazzia VDB, Randt C: Amnesia and eye movements in first stage anesthesia. *Arch Neurol 14:* 522–525, 1966.

Meadow JC: The anatomical basis of prosopagnosia. *J Neurol Neurosurg Psychiat 37:* 489–501, 1974.

Medina JL, Rubino FA, Ross E: Agitated delirium caused by infarction of the hippocampal formation and fusiform and lingual gyri. *Neurology 24:* 1181–1183, 1974.

Meibach RC, Siegel A: Thalamic projections of the hippocampal formation: evidence for an alternate pathway involving the internal capsule. *Brain Res 134:* 1–12, 1977.

Mercer B, Wapner W, Gardner H et al.: A study of confabulation. *Arch Neurol 34:* 429–433, 1977.

Messert B, Wannamaker BB: Reappraisal of the adult occult hydrocephalus syndrome. *Neurology 24:* 224–231, 1974.

Meyer JS, Herndon RM: Bilateral infarction of the pyramidal tracts in man. *Neurology 12:* 637–642, 1962.

Mills RP, Swanson PD: Vertical oculomotor apraxia and memory loss. *Ann Neurol 4:* 149–153, 1978.

Milner B: Brain mechanisms suggested by study of the temporal lobes. In Darley FL and Milliken CH (eds.) *Brain Mechanisms Underlying Speech and Language*, Grune and Stratton, New York, 1967.

Milner B, Taylor L: Right hemisphere superiority in tactile pattern-recognition after cerebral commissurotomy: evidence for nonverbal memory. *Neuropsychol 10:* 1–15, 1972.

Mohr JP, Leicester J, Stoddard LT: Right hemianopsia with memory and color deficits in circumscribed left posterior cerebral artery territory infarction. *Neurology 21:* 1104–1113, 1971.

Mohr JP, Pessin MS, Finkelstein S et al.: Broca aphasia: pathologic and clinical. *Neurology 28:* 311–324, 1978.

Moore MT: Progressive akinetic mutism in cerebellar hemangioblastoma with "normal-pressure hydrocephalus". *Neurology 19:* 32–42, 1969.

Monaco F, Riccio A, Benna P et al. Further observations on carbamazepine plasma levels in epileptic patients. *Neurology 26:* 936–943, 1976.

Moran CMW: *Churchill: The Struggle for Survival, 1940–1965.* Houghton Mifflin, Boston, 1966.

Morgan AH, MacDonald H, Hilgard ER: EEG alpha: lateral asymmetry related to task and hypnotizability. *Psychophysiol 11:* 275–282, 1974.

Morgane PJ, Stern WC: Chemical anantomy of brain circuits in relation to sleep and wakefulness. In Weitzman ED (ed.) *Advances in Sleep Research*, Vol I, Spectrum Pub., New York, 1974.

Morrow LB: How thyroid disease presents in the elderly. *Geriatrics 33:* 42–45, 1978.

Moruzzi G, Magoun HW: Brain stem reticular formation and activation of the electroencephalogram. *Electroenceph Clin Neurophysiol 16:* 2–17, 1949.

Mueller CB: Some effects of health insurance in Canada: from pirvate enterprise toward public accountability. *N Engl J Med 298:* 535–539, 1978.

Muller EE: Nervous control of growth hormone secretion. *Neuroendocrinol 11:* 338–369, 1973.

Muller J, Shaw L: Arterial vascularization of the human hippocampus. *Arch Neurol 13:* 45–47, 1965.

Mumenthaler M: *Neurology* (transl.). Yearbook Medical Pub., Chicago, 1977, p. 2.

Munch-Peterson S, Pakkenberg H, Kornerup H et al.: RNA treatment of dementia: a double-blind study. *Acta Neurol Scandinav 50:* 553–572, 1974.

Muramoto O, Kuru Y, Sugishita M et al.: Pure memory loss with hippocampal lesions. Arch Neurol *36:* 54–56.

Murphy MJ, Lyon LW, Carlstrom TA et al.: Normal pressure hydrocephalus due to membranous obstruction of the sylvian aqueduct. *Neurology 28:* 835–837, 1978.

Murray RM, Greene JG, Adams JH: Analgesic abuse and dementia. *Lancet 3:* 242–245, 1971.

Naeser MA, Hayward RW: Lesion localization in aphasia with cranial computed tomography and the Boston Diagnostic Aphasia Exam. *Neurology 28:* 545–551, 1978.

Nauta WJH: Neural associations of the amygdaloid complex in the monkey. *Brain 85:* 505–520, 1962.

Nebes RD: Perception of spatial relationships by the right and left hemispheres in commissurotomized man. *Neuropsychol 11:* 285–289, 1973.

Nebes RD: Hemispheric specialization in commissurotomized man. *Psychol Bull 8:* 1–14, 1974.

Nebes RD, Sperry RW: Hemispheric deconnection syndrome with cerebral birth injury in the dominant arm area. *Neuropsychol 9:* 247–259, 1971.

Neubauer C: Mental deterioration in epilepsy due to folate deficiency. *Brit Med J 2:* 759–761, 1970.

Neumann MA, Cohn R: Progressive subcortical gliosis, a rare form of presenile dementia. *Brain 90:* 405–418, 1967.

Newton FH, Rosenberg RN, Lampert RW et al.: Neurologic involvement in Urbach-Wiethe's disease (lipoid proteinosis). *Neurology 21:* 1205–1212, 1971.

Norrsell U: Defects in tactile directional sensitivity after forebrain commissurotomizing in man. *Nature 245:* 41–42, 1973.

Obrecht R, Okhomina FOA, Scott DF: Value of EEG in acute confusional states. *J Neurol Neurosurg Psychiat 42:* 75–77, 1979.

Ohya T, Martinez J, Jabbour JT: Subacute sclerosing panencephalitis. Correlation of clinical, neurophysiologic and neuropathologic findings. *Neurology 24:* 211–218, 1974.

Oka H, Jinnai K: Common projection of the motor cortex to the caudate nucleus and the cerebellum. *Exp Brain Res 31:* 31–421, 1978.

Oke A, Keller R, Mefford I: Lateralization of norenpinephrine in human thalamus. *Science 200:* 1411–1413, 1978.

Oldendorf WH: The quest for an image of the brain: a brief historical and technical review of brain imaging techniques. *Neurology 28:* 517–533, 1978.

O'Neill B, Butler AB, Young E et al. Adult-onset GM_2 gangliosidosis. *Neurology 28:* 1117–1123, 1978.

Oppenheimer DR, Newcombe F: Clinical and anatomic findings in a case of auditory agnosia. *Arch Neurol 35:* 712–719, 1978.

Ostertag CB, Mundinger F: Diagnosis of normal pressure hydrocephalus using CT with CSF enhancement. *Neuroradiol 16:* 216–219, 1978.

Osuntokun BO, Bademosi O, Ogunremi K et al.: Neuropsychiatric manifestations of typhoid fever in 959 patients. *Arch Neurol 27:* 7–13, 1972.

Papez JW: A proposed mechanism of emotion. *Arch Neurol Psychiat 38:* 725–734, 1937.

Pattern B: Transient global amnesia syndrome. *J Amer Med Ass 217:* 1205–1212, 1971.

Patterson KE, Lawler E, Rochester SR: Retrograde amnesia from electroconvulsive therapy. *Neuropsychol 16:* 91–97, 1978.

Paulson G, Gottlieb G: Development reflexes: the reappearance of fetal and neonatal reflexes in aged patients. *Brain 91:* 37–52, 1968.

Pender JW: Dissociative anesthesia. *J Amer Med Ass 215:* 1126–1134, 1971.

Pennal BE: Human cerebral asymmetry in color discrimination. *Neuropsychol 15:* 563–568, 1977.

Penry JK, Daly DD (eds.): *Complex Partial Seizures and Their Treatment.* Raven Press, New York, 1975.

Perry TL, Wright JM, Hansen S et al.: Isoniazid therapy of Huntington disease. *Neurology 29:* 370–375, 1979.

Pizzo PA, Bleyer WA, Poplack DG et al.: Reversible dementia temporally associated with intraventricular therapy with methotrexate in a child with acute myelogenous leukemia. *J Pediat 88:* 131–133, 1976.

Plum F: Suppression of oculovestibular responses by depressant drugs. *Arch Neurol 35:* 102–103, 1978.

Plum F, Posner JB: *Stupor and Coma*, 2nd edition. FA Davis, Philadelphia, 1972.

Poeck K, Orgass B: An experimental investigation of finger agnosia. *Neurology 19:* 801–807, 1969.

Porac C, Coren S: The dominant eye. *Psychol Bull 83:* 880–897, 1976.

Porac C, Coren S: The assessment of motor control in sighting dominance using an illusion decrement procedure. *Percep and Psychophys 21:* 631–632, 1977.

Preilowski BFB: Possible contribution of the anterior forebrain commissures to bilateral motor coordination. *Neuropsychol 10:* 267–277, 1972.

Pribram KH: The case for a brain electrodiagnostic in "functional" disorders. In S Bogoch (ed.), *The Biological Diagnosis of Brain Disorders*. Spectrum, New York, 1973.

Puccetti R: Brain bisection and personal identity. *Brit J Philosoph Sci 24:* 339–355, 1973.

Raisman G, Cowan WM, Powell TPS: The extrinsic afferent, commissural and association fibers of the hippocampus. *Brain 88:* 963–996, 1965.

Rao DB, Georgiev EL, Paul PD et al.: Cyclandelate in the treatment of senile mental changes: a double-blind evaluation. *J Amer Geriat Soc 25:* 548–551, 1977.

Ratner J, Rosenberg G, Kral VA et al.: Anticoagulant therapy for senile dementia. *J Amer Geriat Soc 20:* 556–559, 1972.

Raymond RW, Williams RL: Infectious mononucleosis with psychosis. *N Engl J Med 239:* 542–544, 1948.

Reier CE, Hamelberg W: Conscious analgesia and amnesia for cardioversion. *J Amer Med Ass 210:* 2052–2054, 1969.

Reynolds EH, Rothfeld P, Pincus JH: Neurological disease associated with folate deficiency. *Brit Med J 2:* 398–400, 1973.

Rhodes LE, Obitz FW, Creel D: Effect of alcohol and task on hemispheric asymmetry of visually evoked potentials in man. *Electroenceph Clin Neurophysiol 38:* 561–568, 1975.

Rice E, Gendelman S: Psychiatric aspects of normal pressure hydrocephalus. *J Amer Med Ass 223:* 409–412, 1973.

Richardson JC: Principles of diagnosis in neurology. *Can J Neurol Sci 4:* 1–3, 1977.

Riese W: Auto-observation of aphasia: reported by an eminent 19th century medical scientist. *Bull Hist Med 28:* 237–242, 1954.

Riese W: *A History of Neurology*. MD Pub., New York, 1959.

Riese W: Baudelaire as a victim of aphasia. *Episteme 6:* 305–317, 1972.

Riese W: Baudelaire's aphasia. *Neurolinguistics 7:* 25–39, 1977.

Risberg J, Halsey JH, Willis EL et al.: Hemispheric specialization in normal man studied by bilateral measurements of the regional cerebral blood flow: a study with the 133-Xe inhalation technique. *Brain 98:* 511–524, 1975.

Rizzolatti G, Umilta C, Berlucchi G: Opposite superiorities of the right and left cerebral hemispheres in discriminative reaction time to physiognomical and alphabetical material. *Brain 94:* 431–442, 1971.

Robbins KI, McAdam DW: Interhemispheric alpha asymmetry and imagery mode. *Brain Lang 1:* 189–193, 1974.

Rodin EA: Psychosocial management of patients with complex partial seizures. *Adv Neurol 11:* 383–414, 1975.

Romanul FCA, Radvany J, Rosales RK: Whipple's disease confined to the brain: a case studied clinically and pathologically. *J Neurol Neurosurg Psychiat 40:* 901–909, 1977.

Roos D, Willanger R: Various degrees of dementia in a selected group of gastrectomized patients with low serum B_{12}. *Acta Neurol Scandinav 55:* 363–376, 1977.

Rosati G, DeBastiani P: Pure agraphia: a discrete form of aphasia. *J Neurol Neurosurg Psychiat 42:* 266–269, 1979.

Rose HD, Golbert TM, Sanz CJ et al.: Fever during acute alcohol withdrawal. *Amer J Med Sci 260:* 112–121, 1970.

Rosen H, DiGiacomo JR: The role of physical restraint in the treatment of psychiatric illness. *J Clin Psychiat 39:* 228–232, 1978.

Rosenberger PB: Discriminative aspects of visual hemi-inattention. *Neurology 24:* 17–23, 1974.

Rosenzweig MR, Bennett EL: Cerebral changes in rats exposed individually to an enriched environment. *J Comp Physiol Psychol 80:* 304–313, 1972.

Rovit RL, Schecter MM, Ortega B et al.: Progressive ventricular dilatation following pneumoencephalography: a radiological sign of occult hydrocephalus. *J Neurosurg 36:* 50–59, 1972.

Ruble DN: Premenstrual symptoms: a reinterpretation. *Science 197:* 291–292, 1977.

Russell WR, Nathan PW: Traumatic amnesia. *Brain 69:* 280–300, 1946.

Russell WR, Smith A: Post-traumatic amnesia in closed head injury. *Arch Neurol 5:* 4–17, 1961.

Ryback RS: Alcohol amnesia: observations in seven drinking in-patient alcoholics. *Quant J Stud Alcoh 31:* 616–632, 1970.

Sagan C: *The Dragons of Eden.* Random House, New York, 1977.

Salguero LF, Itabashi HH, Gutierrez NB: Childhood multiple sclerosis with psychotic manifestations. *J Neurol Neurosurg Psychiat 32:* 572–579, 1969.

Salmon JH: Adult hydrocephalus. *J Neurosurg 37:* 423–428, 1972.

Salum I: Delirium tremens and certain other acute sequels of alcohol abuse. *Acta Psychiat Scandinav Suppl 235:* 1–145, 1972.

Sarhaddi S, Bravo E, Curs AE: Gliomatosis cerebri. *Southern Med J 66:* 883–888, 1973.

Sasanuma S: Kana and kanji processing in Japanese aphasics. *Brain Lang 2:* 369–383, 1975.

Savoldi F, Nappi G, Martignoni E et al.: Brain phospholipids in the treatment of chronic cerebrovascular insufficiency. *Curr Therap Res 24:* 209–226, 1978.

Schacter DL, Crovitz HF: Memory function after closed head injury: a review of the quantitative research. *Cortex 13:* 150–176, 1977.

Schaumburg HH, Suzuki K: Non-specific familial presenile dementia. *J Neurol Neurosurg Psychiat 31:* 479–486, 1968.

Scheibel ME, Scheibel AB: Structural substrates for integrative patterns in the brain stem reticular core. In Jasper HH and Proctor LL (eds.). *Reticular Formation of the Brain.* Little, Brown, Boston, 1958.

Scheibel ME, Scheibel AB: Structural organization of non-specific thalamic nuclei and their projection toward cortex. *Brain Res 6:* 60–94, 1967.

Schentag JJ, Cerra FB, Calleri G et al.: Pharmacokinetic and clinical studies in patients with cimetidine-associated mental confusion. *Lancet 1:* 177–181, 1979.

Schoenberg M, Miller MG, Schoenberg CE: The mind-body dichotomy reified: an illustrative case. *Amer J Psychiat 135:* 1224–1226, 1978.

Schuell H, Jenkins JJ, Jimenez-Pabon E: *Aphasia in Adults: Diagnosis, Prognosis, and Treatment.* Harper Row, New York, 1964.

Schuster MM, Iber FL: Psychosis with pancreatitis. *Arch Int Med 116:* 228–233, 1965.

Scoville WB, Milner B: Loss of recent memory after bilateral hippocampal lesions. *J Neurol Neurosurg Psychiat 20:* 11–21, 1957.

Segarra JM: Cerebral vascular disease and behavior I: the syndrome of the mesencephalic artery. *Arch Neurol 22:* 408–418, 1970.

Seigel A, Ohgami S, Edinger H: Projections of the hippocampus to the septal area in the squirrel monkey. *Brain Res 99:* 247–260, 1975.

Seigman AW: The meaning of silent pauses in the initial interview. *J Nerv Ment Dis 166:* 642–654, 1978.

Serby M, Angrist B, Lieberman A: Mental disturbances during bromocriptine and lergotrile treatment of Parkinson's disease. *Amer J Psychiat 135:* 1227–1229, 1978.

Shem S: *The House of God.* Marek Pub., New York, 1978, p. 37.

Shenkin HA, Crowley JN: Hydrocephalus complicating pituitary adenoma. *J Neurol Neurosurg Psychiat 36:* 479–486, 1973.

Shenken HA, Greenberg J, Bouzarth WF et al.: Ventricular shunting for relief of senile symptoms. *J Amer Med Ass 225:* 1486–1489, 1973.

Shepherd GM: Synaptic organization of the mammalian olfactory bulb. *Physiol Rev 52:* 864–917, 1972.

Shoulson I, Fahn S: Huntington disease: clinical care and evaluation. *Neurology 29:* 1–3, 1979.

Shraberg D: The myth of pseudodementia: depression and the aging brain. *Amer J Psychiat 135:* 601–603, 1978.

Shraberg D, Weisberg L: The Kluver-Bucy syndrome in man. *J Nerv Ment Dis 166:* 130–134, 1978.

Shucard DW, Shucard JL, Thomas DG: Auditory evoked potentials as probes of hemispheric differences in cognitive processing. *Sciences 197:* 1295–1298, 1977.

Shulman R: Psychiatric aspects of pernicious anaemia: a prospective controlled investigation. *Brit Med J 3*: 266–270, 1967.

Shuttleworth EC, Morris CE: The transient global amnesia syndrome: a defect in the second stage of memory in man. *Arch Neurol 15:* 505–520, 1966.

Shuttleworth EC, Wise GR: Transient global amnesia due to arterial embolism. *Arch Neurol 29:* 340–342, 1973.

Silverman D: Some observations on the EEG in hepatic coma. *Electroenceph Clin Neurophysiol 14:* 53–59, 1962.

Sjaastad O, Nornes H: Increased intracranial pressure in so-called "normal-pressure hydrocephalus". *Eur Neurol 14:* 161–177, 1976.

Slater R, Reivichm M, Goldberg H et al.: Diaschisis with cerebral infarction. *Stroke 8:* 684–690, 1977.

Small JG, Milstein V, Stevens JR: Are psychomotor epileptics different? *Arch Neurol 7:* 187–194, 1962.

Smith DA: Nutritional neuropathies in the civilian interment camp, Hong Kong, January, 1942, to August, 1945. *Brain 69:* 209–222, 1946.

Smith DL Jr: Mental effect of mercury poisoning. *Southern Med J 71:* 904–905, 1978.

Smith JS, Brandon S: Morbidity from acute carbon monoxide poisoning at three-year follow-up. *Brit Med J 1:* 318–321, 1973.

Smith JS, Kiloh LG, Ratnavale GS et al.: The investigation of dementia: the results of 100 consecutive admissions. *Med J Austral 2:* 403–405, 1976.

Snowdon JA, MacFie AC, Pearce JB: Hypocalcaemic myopathy with paranoid psychosis. *J Neuro Neurosurg Psychiat 39:* 48–52, 1976.

Snyder BD, Harris S: Treatable aspects of the dementia syndrome. *J Amer Geriat Soc 24:* 179–184, 1976.

Sourander P, Walinder J: Hereditary multi-infarct dementia: morphological and clinical studies of a new disease. *Acta Neuropathol 39:* 247–254, 1977.

Spehlman R, Stahl SM: Dopamine acetylcholine imbalance in Parkinson's disease: possible regenerative overgrowth of cholinergic axon terminals. *Lancet 2:* 724–726, 1976.

Spreen O, Benton AL, VanAllen MW: Dissociation of visual and tactile naming in amnesic aphasia. *Neurology 16:* 807–814, 1966.

Sprofkin BE, Sciarra D: Korsakoff's psychosis associated with cerebral tumors. *Neurology 2:* 427–434, 1952.

Squire LR: A stable impairment in remote memory following electroconvulsive therapy. *Neuropsychol 13:* 51–58, 1975.

Squire LR, Chase PM: Memory functions six to nine months after electroconvulsive therapy. *Arch Gen Psychiat 32:* 1557–1564, 1975.

Squire LR, Slater PC: Anterograde and retrograde memory impairment in chronic amnesia. *Neuropsychol 16:* 313–322, 1978.

State v Jack Ruby: Trial transcript. *Trauma 6:* 5–268, 1964.

Stein JA, Tschudy DP: Acute intermittent porphria. *Medicine 49:* 1–16, 1970.

Stein SC, Langfitt TW: Normal-pressure hydrocephalus. *J Neurosurg 41:* 463–470, 1974.

Stern FH: Management of chronic brain syndrome secondary to cerebral arteriosclerosis with special reference to papaverine hydrochloride. *J Amer Geriat Soc 18:* 507–512, 1970.

Stevens JR: Interictal clinical manifestations of complex partial seizures. *Adv Neurol 11:* 85–112, 1975.

Stevens JR, Milstein V, Goldstein S: Psychomotor test performance in relation to the psychopathology of epilepsy. *Arch Gen Psychiat 26:* 532–538, 1972.

Stigsby B, Risberg J, Ingvar DH: Electroencephalographic changes in the dominant hemisphere during memorising and reasoning. *Electroenceph Clin Neurophysiol 42:* 665–675, 1977.

Stones MJ: Electroconvulsive treatment and short term memory. *Brit J Psychiat 122:* 591–594, 1973.

Strub RL, Black FW: *The Mental Status Examination in Neurology.* FA Davis, Philadelphia, 1977, p. 11.

Stuss DT, Alexander MP, Lieberman A et al.: An extraordinary form of confabulation. *Neurology 28:* 1166–1172, 1978.

Subczynski JA: State of consciousness scoring system. *J Neurol 43:* 251–252, 1975.

Sugar HS, Goldstein AS: Visual anosgnosia in cortical blindness: Anton's syndrome. *Amer J Ophth 60:* 335–337, 1965.

Sutton NR, Singer M: Successful treatment in a woman with Down's syndrome. *Psychiat Opinion 16:* 36–40, 1979.

Suzuki K, David E, Kutschman B: Presenile dementia with "Lafora-like" intraneuronal inclusions. *Arch Neurol 25:* 69–80, 1971.

Symon L, Dorsch NWC: Pressure waves in so-called low-pressure hydrocephalus. *Lancet 4:* 1291–1292, 1972.

Symonds C: Disorders of memory. *Brain 89:* 624–644, 1966.

Sypert GW, Leffman H, Ojemann GA: Occult normal pressure hydrocephalus manifested by parkinsonism-dementia complex. *Neurology 23:* 234–238, 1973.

Teasdale G, Knill-Jones R, Van der Sande J: Observer variability in assessing impaired consciousness and coma. *J Neurol Neurosurg Psychiat 41:* 603–610, 1978.

Teece JJ: Contingent negative variation and individual differences: a new approach in brain research. *Arch Gen Psychiat 24:* 1–16, 1971.

Teng EL, Sperry RW: Interhemispheric interaction during simultaneous bilateral presentation of letters or digits in commisurotomized patients. *Neuropsychol 11:* 131–140, 1973.

Terzian H, Dalle Ore G: Syndrome of Kluver and Bucy reproduced in man by bilateral removal of the temporal lobes. *Neurology 5:* 373–380, 1955.

Theander S, Granholm L: Sequelae after spontaneous subarachnoid haemorrhage, with special reference to hydrocephalus and Korsakoff's syndrome. *Acta Neurol Scandinav 43:* 479–488, 1967.

Thomas FB, Mazzaferri EL, Skillman TG: Apathetic thyrotoxicosis: a distinctive clinical and laboratory entity. *Ann Int Med 72:* 679–685, 1970.

Thompson GL: Cerebral lesions simulating schizophrenia: three case reports. *Biol Psychiat 2:* 59–64, 1970.

Thompson GN: The electroencephalogram in acute pathological alcoholic intoxication. *Bull LA Neurol Soc 28:* 217–224, 1963.

Thompson WL, Johnson AD, Maddrey WL et al.: Diazepam and paraldehyde for treatment of severe delirium tremens. *Ann Int Med 82:* 175–180, 1975.

Thomson AD, Baker H, Leevy CM: Patterns of S^{35}-thiamine hydrochloride absorption in the malnourished alcoholic patient. *J Lab Clin Med 76:* 34–45, 1970.

Thornton WE: Dementia induced by methyldopa with haloperidol. *N Engl J Med 295:* 1222, 1976.

Tindall RSA, Willerson J: Subacute phenytoin intoxication syndrome. *Arch Int Med 138:* 1168–1169, 1978.

Todorov AB, Go RCP, Constantinidis J et al.: Specificity of the clinical diagnosis of dementia. *J Neurol Sci 26:* 81–98, 1975.

Tomlinson BE, Walton JN: Superficial haemosiderosis of the central nervous system. *J Neurol Neurosurg Psychiat 27:* 332–339, 1964.

Tonali P, Laudisio A, Belloni G et al.: Functional obstructive hydrocephalus. *Neuroradiol 5:* 220–222, 1973.

Torack RM, Hughes CP: Neuroaxonal dystrophy in subacute dementia. *Acta Neuropath 22*: 264–268, 1972.

Torrey EF: What is the future of psychiatry as a medical speciality? Bleak at best. In Brodie JP, Brodie HKH (eds.), *Controversy in Psychiatry*, Saunders, Philadelphia, 1978.

Torvik A, Dietrichson P, Svaar H et al.: Myopathy with tremor and dementia: A metabolic disorder? *J Neurol Sci 21:* 181–190, 1974.

Trapp GA, Miner GD, Zimmerman RL et al.: Aluminum levels in brain in Alzheimer's disease. *Biol Psychiat 13:* 709-718, 1978.

Trevarthen C, Sperry RW: Perceptual unity of the ambient visual field in human commissurotomy patients. *Brain 96:* 547–570, 1973.

Trost JE, Canter GJ: Apraxia of speech in patients with Broca's aphasia: a study of phoneme production accuracy and error patterns. *Brain Lang 1:* 63–79, 1974.

Trotter JL, Luzecky M, Siegel BA et al.: Cerebrospinal fluid infusion test. *Neurology 24:* 181–186, 1974.

Troupin A, Ojemann LM, Halpren L et al: Carbamazepine: a double-blind comparison with phenytoin. *Neurology 27:* 511–519, 1977.

Tucker DM, Watson RT, Heilman KM: Discrimination and evocation of affectively intoned speech in patients with right parietal disease. *Neurology 27:* 947–950, 1977.

Tylden E: Bromism. *Lancet 4:* 924, 1971.

Vallarta JM, Bell DB, Reichert A: Progressive encephalopathy due to chronic hydantoin intoxication. *Amer J Dis Child 128:* 27–34, 1974.

Van Buren JM, Borke RC: The mesial temporal substratum of memory: anatomical studies in three individuals. *Brain 95:* 599–632, 1972.

Van Hosen GW, Pandya, DN, Butters N: Cortical afferents to the entorhinal cortex of the rhesus monkey. *Science 175:* 1471–1473, 1972.

Van Putten T, Menkes JH: Huntington's disease masquerading as chronic schizophrenia. *Dis Nerv Syst 34:* 54–56, 1973.

Vetter WR, Cohn LH, Reichgott M: Hypokalemia and electrocardiographic abnormalities during acute alcohol withdrawal. *Arch Int Med 120:* 536–541, 1967.

Victor M, Adams RD: The effect of alcohol on the nervous system. *Assoc Nerv Ment Dis 32:* 526–573, 1953.

Victor M, Adams RD, Collins GH: *The Wernicke-Korsakoff Syndrome.* FA Davis, Philadelphia, 1971.

Victor M, Angevine JB, Mancall EI et al.: Memory loss with lesions of hippocampal formation: report of a case with some remarks on the anatomical of memory. *Arch Neurol 5:* 244–263, 1961.

Victor M, Brausch C: The role of abstinence in the genesis of alcoholic epilepsy. *Epilepsia 8:* 1–20, 1967.

Vincent FM, Sadowsky CH, Saunders RL et al.: Alexia without agraphia, hemianopia, or color-naming defect: a disconnection syndrome. *Neurology 27:* 689–691, 1977.

Wall PD: The gate control theory of pain mechanisms. *Brain 101:* 1–18, 1978.

Walton JN: *Brain's Diseases of the Nervous System*, 8th ed. Oxford University Press, New York, 1977.

Watson RT, Heilman KM: Thalamic neglect. *Neurology 29:* 690–694, 1979.

Watson RT, Heilman KM, Cauthen JC et al.: Neglect after cingulectomy. *Neurology 23:* 1003–1007, 1973.

Watson RT, Heilman KM, Miller BD et al.: Neglect after mesencephalic reticular formation lesions. *Neurology 24:* 294–298, 1974.

Watson RT, Miller BD, Heilman KM: Nonsensory neglect. *Ann Neurol 3:* 505–508, 1978.

Waxman SG, Geschwind N: Hypergraphia in temporal lobe epilepsy. *Neurology 24:* 629–636, 1974.

Waxman SG, Geschwind N: The interictal behavior syndrome of temporal lobe epilepsy. *Arch Gen Psychiat 32:* 1580–1586, 1975.

Webster WG: Territoriality and the evolution of brain asymmetry. *Ann NY Acad Sci 299:* 213–221, 1977.

Weindl A: Neuroendocrine aspects of circumventricular organs. In *Frontiers in Neuroendocrinology*, Ganong WF and Martini L (eds.), Oxford University Press, New York, 1973.

Weinstein EA, Friedland RP: Behavioral disorders associated with hemi-inattention. *Adv Neurol 18:* 61–62, 1977.

Weinstein EA, Friedland RP (eds.): *Hemi-Inattention and Hemisphere Specialization.* Raven, New York, 1977.

Weiskrantz L: Behavioral analysis of the monkey's visual nervous system. *Proc R Soc Lond 182:* 427–455, 1972.

Wells CE: *Dementia*, 2nd ed, FA Davis, Philadelphia, 1977.

Wells CE: Pseudodementia. *Amer J Psychiat 136:* 895–900, 1979.

Wernicke C: The aphasia symptom-complex: a psychological study on an anatomical basis. *Arch Neurol 22:* 280–282, 1874 (transl. 1970).

Wertheim N: The amusias. In Vinken PJ, Bruyn GW (eds.), *Disorders of Higher Nervous Activity*, Vol. 4 of *Handbook of Clinical Neurology*, North Holland Pub. Co., Amsterdam, 1964.

Westmoreland BF, Klass DW, Sharbrough FW et al. Alpha coma. *Arch Neurol 32:* 713–718, 1975.

White P, Hiley CR, Goodhardt MJ et al.: Neocortical cholinergic neurons in elderly people. *Lancet 1:* 668–671, 1977.

Whitley RJ, Soong SJ, Dolin R et al.: Adenosine arabinoside therapy of biopsy-proved herpes simplex encephalitis. *N Engl J Med 297:* 289–294, 1977.

Whittaker H: A case of isolation of the speech area. In Whittaker H and Whittaker HA (eds.), *Studies in Neurolinguistics 2:* Academic Press, New York, 1976.

Whittaker HA, Ojemann GA: Graded localization of naming from electrical stimulation mapping of left cerebral cortex. *Nature 270:* 50–51, 1977.

Whitty CWM, Lewin W: A Korsakoff syndrome in the post-cingulectomy confusional state. *Brain 83:* 648–653, 1960.

Williams JA, Hall GS, Thompson AG et al.: Neurological disease after partial gastrectomy. *Brit Med J 3:* 210–212, 1969.

Williams M, Smith HV: Mental disturbances in tuberculous meningitis. *J Neurol Neurosurg Psychiat 17:* 173–182, 1954.

Wilson DL: On the nature of consciousness and of physical reality. *Persp Biol Med 19:* 568–581, 1976.

Wilson LG: Viral encephalopathy mimicking functional psychosis. *Amer J Psychiat 133:* 165–169, 1976.

Winner E, Gardner H: The comprehension of metaphor in brain damaged patients. *Brain 100:* 717–729, 1977.
Wintrob RM: Malaria and the acute psychotic episode. *J Nerv Ment Dis 156:* 306–317, 1973.
Wisniewski K, Jervis GA, Moretz RC et al.: Alzheimer neurofibrillary tangles in diseases other than senile and presenile disease. *Ann Neurol 5:* 288–294, 1978.
Wolf SM: Difficulties in right-left discrimination in a normal population. *Arch Neurol 29:* 128–129, 1973.
Wolinsky JS, Barnes BD, Margolis MT: Diagnostic tests in normal pressure hydrocephalus. *Neurology 23:* 706–713, 1973.
Yakovlev PJ, Koskoss DY, Patton RA: Limbic nuclei of thalamus and connections of limbic cortex I: organization of the projections of the anterior group of nuclei and of the midline nuclei of the thalamus to the anterior cingulate gyrus and hippocampal rudiment of the monkey. *Arch Neurol 3:* 620–641, 1960.
Yamadori A, Osumi Y, Masuhara S et al.: Preservation of singing in Broca's aphasia. *J Neurol Neurosurg Psychiat 40:* 221–224, 1977.
Yarnell PR, Lynch S: Retrograde memory immediately after concussion. *Lancet 1:* 863–864, 1970.
Yarnell PR, Lynch S: The "ding": amnestic states in football trauma. *Neurology 23:* 196–197, 1973.
Yesavage JA, Tinklenberg JR, Hollister LE et al.: Vasodilators in senile dementias: a review of the literature. *Arch Gen Psychiat 36:* 220–223, 1979.
Yoshii N: Follow-up study of epileptic patients following Forel-H-tomy. *Appl Neurophysiol 40:* 1–12, 1977.
Zaidel D, Sperry RW: Memory impairment after commissurotomy in man. *Brain 97:* 263–272, 1974.
Zervas NT, Hedley-White J: Successful treatment of cerebral herniation in five patients. *N Engl J Med 286:* 1075–1077, 1972.
Ziegler DK, Kaufman A, Marshall HE: Abrupt memory loss associated with thalamic tumor. *Arch Neurol 34:* 545–548, 1977.

Supplemental Bibliography

Ashford JW, Schulz SC, Walsh GO: Violent automatism in a partial complex seizure. *Arch Neurol 37:* 120–121, 1980.

Berger EY: A system for rating the severity of senility. *J Amer Geriat Soc 28:* 234–236, 1980.

Bergman H, Borg S, Holm L: Neuropsychological impairment and exclusive abuse of sedatives or hypnotics. *Amer J Psychiat 137:* 215–217, 1980.

Black PM: Idiopathic normal-pressure hydrocephalus. Results of shunting in 62 patients. *J Neurosurg 52:* 371–377, 1980.

Boller F, Mizutani T, Roessman U et al.: Parkinson disease, dementia, and Alzheimer disease: Clinicopathological correlations. *Ann Neurol 7:* 329–335, 1979.

Brust JCM: Music and language: Musical alexia and agraphia. *Brain 103:* 367–372, 1980.

Byer JA, Crowley WJ: Musical performance during transient global amnesia. *Neurology 30:* 80–82, 1980.

Cotman CW, McGaugh JL: *Behavioral Neuroscience.* Academic Press, New York, 838p., 1980.

Damasio AR, Chui HC, Corbett J et al.: Posterior callosal section in a non-epileptic patient. *J Neurol Neurosurg Psychiat 43:* 351–356, 1980.

Damasio H, Damasio AR: The anatomical basis of conduction aphasia. *Brain 103:* 337–342, 1980.

DeRenzi E, Motti F, Nichelli P: Imitating gestures. A quantitative approach to ideomotor apraxia. *Arch Neurol 37:* 6–10, 1980.

Dimond SJ: *Neuropsychology.* Butterworths, London, 560pp., 1980.

Earnest MP, Heaton RK, Wilkinson WE et al.: Cortical atrophy, ventricular enlargement and intellectual impairment in the aged. *Neurology 29:* 1138–1143, 1979.

Glick SD, Weaver LM, Meibach RC: Lateralization of reward in rats: Differences in reinforcing thresholds. *Science 207:* 1093–1095, 1980.

Heilman KM, Valenstein E: *Clinical Neuropsychology.* 674pp., 1979.

Hermann BP, Schwartz MS, Karnes WE et al.: Psychopathology in epilepsy: Relationship of seizure type to age at onset. *Epilepsia 21:* 15–23, 1979.

Hetnarski B, Wisniewski HM, Iqbal K et al.: Central cholinergic activity in aluminum-induced neurofibrillary degeneration. *Ann Neurol 7:* 489–490, 1980.

Hier DB, Caplan LR: Drugs for senile dementia. *Drugs 20:* 74–80, 1980.

Jensen TS, Olivarius BD: Transient global amnesia as a manifestation of transient cerebral ischemia. *Acta Neurol Scandinav 61:* 115–123, 1980.

Johnston RB, Mellits ED: Pediatric coma: Prognosis and outcome. *Develop Med Child Neurol 22:* 3–12, 1980.

Kapur N, Coughlan AK: Confabulation and frontal lobe dysfunction. *J. Neurol Neurosurg Psychiat 43:* 461–463, 1980.

Kaszniak AW, Garron DC, Fox JH et al.: Cerebral atrophy, EEG slowing, age, education, and cognitive functioning in suspected dementia. *Neurology 29:* 1273–1279, 1979.

Knopman DS, Rubens AB, Klassen AC et al.: Regional cerebral blood flow patterns during verbal and nonverbal auditory activation. *Brain Lang 9:* 93–112, 1980.

Levin HS, O'Donnell VM, Grossman RG: The Galveston orientation and amnesia test. A practical scale to assess cognition after head injury. *J Nerv Ment Dis 167:* 675–684, 1979.

Levine DN, Calvanio R: Visual discrimination after lesion of the posterior corpus callosum. *Neurology 30:* 21–30, 1980.

Lipowski ZJ: A new look at organic brain syndrome. *Amer J Psychiat 137:* 674–678, 1980.

Lipowski ZJ: *Delirium. Acute Brain Failure in Man.* Charles C. Thomas, Springfield, IL 567pp., 1980.

Maltbie AA, Wingfield MS, Volow MR et al.: Electroconvulsive therapy in the presence of brain tumor. *J Nerv Ment Dis 168:* 400–405, 1980.

Mayexu R, Brandt J, Rosen J et al.: Interictal memory and language impairment in temporal lobe epilepsy. *Neurology 30:* 120–125, 1980.

McEntee WJ, Mair RB: Memory enhancement in Korsakoff's psychosis by clonidine: Further evidence for a noradrenergic deficit. *Ann Neurol 7:* 466–470, 1980.

Meudell PR, Northen B: Long term memory for famous voices in amnesic and normal subjects. *Neuropsychologia 18:* 133–139, 1980.

Moraiu MA: Progressive supranuclear palsy and normal pressure hydrocephalus. *Neurology 29:* 1544–1546, 1979.

Mumenthaler M, Kaesar HE, Hess T; Transient global amnesia after clioquinol: Five personal observations from outside Japan. *J Neurol Neurosurg Psychiat 42:* 1084–1090, 1979.

Petit TL, Biederman GB, McMullen PA: Neurofibrillary degeneration, dendritic dying back, and learning-memory deficits after aluminum administration: Implications for brain aging. *Exper Neurol 67:* 152–162, 1980.

Perl DP, Brody AR: Alzheimer's disease: X-ray spectrometric evidence of aluminum accumulation in neurofibrillary tangle-bearing neurons. *Science 208:* 297–299, 1980.

Pincus JH: Can violence be a manifestation of epilepsy? *Neurology 30:* 304–307, 1980.

Platt FW, McMath JC: Clinical hypocompetence: The interview. *Ann Int Med 91:* 898–902, 1979.

Ponsford JL, Donnan GA: Transient global amnesia: A hippocampal phenomenon? *J Neurol Neurosurg Psychiat 43:* 285–287, 1980.

Rosen WG, Terry RD, Fuld PA et al.: Pathological verification of ischemic score in differentiation of dementias. *Ann Neurol 7:* 486–488, 1980.

Robinson RG, Coyle JT: The differential effect of right versus left hemispheric cerebral infarction on catecholamines and behavior in the rat. *Brain Res 188:* 63–78, 1980.

Ross ED: Sensory-specific and fractional disorders of recent memory in man. *Arch Neurol 37:* 193–200, 1980.

Ruben I, Wolkon G, Yamamoto J: Physical attacks on psychiatric residents by patients. *J Nerv Ment Dis 168:* 243–245, 1980.

Ruff RL, Russakoff LM: Catatonia with frontal lobe atrophy. *J Neurol Neurosurg Psychiat 43:* 185–187, 1980.

Santos AB, McCurdy L: Delirium after abrupt withdrawal from doxepin: Case report. *Amer J Psychiat 137:* 239–240, 1980.

Schwartz AS, Marchok PL, Kreinick et al.: The asymmetric lateralization of tactile extinction in patients with unilateral cerebral dysfunction. *Brain 102:* 669–684, 1979.

Taylor MA, Abrams R, Faber R et al.: Cognitive tasks in the mental status examination. *J Nerv Ment Dis 168:* 167–170, 1980.

Wetzel CD, Squire LR: Encoding in anterograde amnesia. *Neuropsychologia 18:* 177–184, 1980.

Wolraich ML, Reiter S: Training physicians in communication skills. *Develop Med Child Neurol 21:* 773–778.

Yagishita S, Itoh Y, Amano N et al.: Atypical senile dementia with widespread Lewy type inclusion in the cerebral cortex. *Acta Neuropathol 49:* 187–191, 1980.

Yamada F, S Fukuda, Samejima et al.: Significance of pathognomonic features of normal-pressure hydrocephalus on computerized tomography. *Neuroradiol 16:* 212–213, 1978.

Index

GPSR Compliance

The European Union's (EU) General Product Safety Regulation (GPSR) is a set of rules that requires consumer products to be safe and our obligations to ensure this.

If you have any concerns about our products, you can contact us on ProductSafety@springernature.com

In case Publisher is established outside the EU, the EU authorized representative is:

Springer Nature Customer Service Center GmbH
Europaplatz 3
69115 Heidelberg, Germany

Batch number: 10607212

Printed by Printforce, the Netherlands